How to Examine the Nervous System

T0180179

How to Examine the Nervous System

fourth edition

R. T. Ross
Member of the Order of Canada
Doctor of Medicine and Doctor of Science of the University of Manitoba
Fellow of the Royal College of Physicians of London
Fellow of the Royal College of Physicians and Surgeons of Canada
Emeritus Professor of Medicine, Section of Neurology
University of Manitoba, Health Sciences Centre
Winnipeg, Canada

With a Foreword by
Lewis P. Rowland, MD
Columbia University Medical Center,
New York

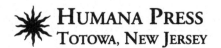

HUMANA PRESS
TOTOWA, NEW JERSEY

This book is dedicated to the memory and influences of two men:

J.D. Adamson, MD (Manitoba), MRCP (Edinburgh), FRCP (Canada), Professor and Chairman, Department of Medicine, University of Manitoba, 1939–1951

L.G. Bell, OC, MBE, MD (Manitoba), LLD (Queens University, Kingston, Ontario), FRCP (London and Canada), FACP, Professor and Chairman, Department of Medicine, University of Manitoba, 1951–1964

I had the good luck to be taught by both of these doctors. J.D. Adamson could take a better history and elicit more information from a patient than anyone I have ever met. He considered every new patient a fascinating story-teller. He asked few questions, managed to keep the patient on the subject, and was completely enthralled as the history unwound. He knew the words and music of disease.

L.G. Bell could see more in 10 seconds at the bedside and do a better physical examination than anyone else. He had a great ability to find, see, and feel (or maybe smell) abnormal physical signs. One learned as much from watching him examine as from listening to J.D. Adamson listen.

Both of these men taught hundreds of students, interns, and residents. Each had great respect for the skills of the other. They were cultured, well-read, humorous humans and great bedside doctors who dearly loved medicine and teaching.

> A man does not learn to understand anything unless he loves it.—Goethe

Contents

Foreword

Robert T. Ross is one of the most respected neurologists in North America. He established and led the Department of Neurology at the University of Manitoba for many years. He founded the *Canadian Journal of Neurological Sciences* in 1974 and was editor-in-chief until 1981. He has written and published 88 papers on clinical problems in neurology. He has been made an Honorary Life Member of the Canadian Neurological Society and was given an Honorary Degree by the University of Manitoba. He has also been awarded the Order of Canada.

Dr. Ross knows how to examine patients and he knows how to teach medical students, especially those who are just beginning to learn neurology. They are the ones most likely to be perplexed by the apparent complexity of the neurological examination. Dr. Ross has come to their rescue with this book.

With simple and direct writing, and numerous illustrations that serve the purpose, he shows that examination is not all that difficult, that it can make sense, and that it can be done in a few minutes. Once the student feels some confidence, the examination can bring pleasure and a sense of achievement. The student then becomes part of the health care team in support of the patients.

Dr. Ross' skilled exposition has made the first three editions of this book a success and it has been the recommended text in many medical schools. Any book that has gone through three editions must be on the right track, and this fourth edition keeps up the pace.

Lewis P. Rowland, MD
Neurological Institute
Columbia University Medical Center
New York, NY

Preface

> The more resources we have, the more complex they are, the greater are the demands upon our clinical skill. These resources are calls upon judgment and not substitutes for it. Do not, therefore, scorn clinical examination; learn it sufficiently to get from it all it holds, and gain in the confidence it merits.
>
> —Sir Francis Walshe, 1952

Technical advances have made diagnoses quicker, safer, and more accurate. Sometimes it appears that careful history taking and examination are less important than knowing which test to order.

However, the technology is expensive and access is limited. As medical costs are increasingly scrutinized by the paying agencies, private or public, there will be limitations on both diagnostic investigations and hospital admissions.

For patients and doctors in smaller centers, limitations already exist. These conditions make a careful history and examination essential to the intelligent care of the sick and prerequisites for ordering tests. The practice of diagnostic medicine is not simply 'scene' recognition plus knowing where to point the technology. If it ever becomes this, a clerk—and eventually a machine—will be able to do it. Therefore, I suggest that you learn how to listen to and examine patients thoroughly and confidently. It is the most precious and durable skill you have; the more you use it, the better it becomes. It is unique.

> One learns by doing the thing; for though you think you know it, you have no certainty until you try.
>
> —Sophocles

In the examination of sick people a *technique* that elicits physical signs, and the ability to *interpret* those signs, are required.

Interpreting physical signs is one of the interesting parts of neurology. The process will not work if abnormal signs have been missed because of faulty technique, or if minor variations within the limits of normal are considered as firm abnormalities. Each year more students must be taught more subjects as the knowledge explosion continues. Only a small amount of time can be spent on the method of any physical examination. Therefore, learn a reliable technique quickly.

This book offers some anatomical and a smaller number of pathological possibilities that may explain a physical sign. It does not consist of a list of, for example, all the possible causes of an absent corneal reflex, and is *not* a small textbook of neurological diseases.

Teach and be taught is a ground rule that most of us will try to observe all of our professional lives. Every doctor and medical student owes a debt to *patients*, who are an essential part of the teaching situation. They allow us to teach 'on' them and around them, and they tolerate several history takings and physical examinations, usually for the benefit of someone else.

At all times one must treat patients with respect and kindness. When you enter the room, identify yourself and tell the patient why you are there. Do not persist with the history or examination past the point at which the patient is tired or uncooperative. Patients are most cooperative with students and doctors who are clean, neat, and polite.

When examining a patient, stand on the right side of the bed (or on the left if you are left-handed). After you have identified yourself, level the bed; that is, if the head or knee break is cranked up, flatten it. Then raise the bed as high as it will go. You can work better with the bed 30 inches from the floor.

Spend 60–75% of the time devoted to any one patient on history taking and the remainder on the physical examination. Have a system of examination and learn to follow it in the same way each time.

Do not be upset by the transient nature of some physical signs. You may see a patient with a slightly enlarged left pupil and explosively hyperactive tendon reflexes in the right arm and leg and a right extensor plantar response. Examination a short while later shows that the pupils and tendon reflexes are equal and both plantar responses are flexor. Both examinations were valid. Few physical signs of acute diseases of the nervous system are fixed. Papilledema is a notable exception. If it was present yesterday, it will be there today, tomorrow, and the day after. Almost all other signs can change hourly or daily.

R. T. Ross, CM, MD, DSc, FRCP

Acknowledgments

It is a pleasure to acknowledge and thank the people who have contributed to this book.

Gail Landry has done some artwork, posed as a model for the illustrations, and typed the manuscript several times.

Angela Ross has read and reread the manuscript for English, grammar, and syntax.

Drs. A.C. Huntington and A.J. Gomori have reviewed and edited the ophthalmology and other portions of the second edition and their suggestions have been included in the current edition. Dr. David Steven has acted as a model for some illustrations. I am grateful to these three physicians.

Rob Mathieson has skillfully photographed parts of the examination, and Cameron Walker has done all the drawings.

The Ophthalmoscope, the Fundus Oculi, and Central and Peripheral Vision

1

The examination of the eye consists of five parts. This chapter deals with the fundus oculi and with central and peripheral vision. The remaining three parts of the examination are described in later chapters.

THE OPHTHALMOSCOPE

There are five mechanical details you need to know about the head of the ophthalmoscope. The following remarks apply to the Welch-Allyn ophthalmoscope (Figure 1–1).

Buy an ophthalmoscope with a halogen bulb and handle that takes D-size batteries. A handle containing a rechargeable cell is almost as big as the D-size battery model and just as good. The ophthalmoscope that takes AA batteries is undesirable. The power does not last long enough, and the scope is difficult to hold.

When you attach the head to the handle, have the on-off button in front, as in Figure 1–1. To turn it on, push in the on-off button and turn the disc that contains it. It turns only one way. As you rotate the lens selector wheel, the numbers change in the lens strength window. This changes the amount of magnification between your eye and the patient's retina when you are looking through the viewing aperture. If the lens selector wheel is turned clockwise in the direction of the heavy arrow, increasingly stronger plus lenses continue to appear in the viewing aperture and increasingly higher black numbers continue to appear in the lens strength window. On the back of the ophthalmoscope there is another adjustable wheel, the aperture selector, which rotates in a horizontal plane. You will find that rotating this wheel produces a green circle, a large white circle, a small white circle, or a grid. Turn it back to the large white circle and leave it there. (If the white circles appear orange, get new batteries, and if still orange, get a new bulb.)

1

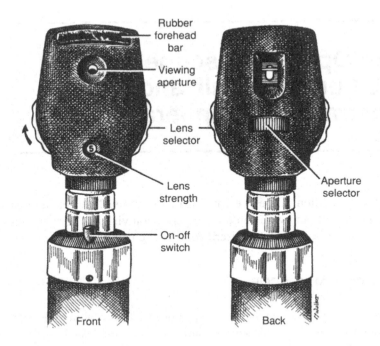

Figure 1–1. Details of the ophthalmoscope head (Welch-Allyn).

THE FUNDUS OCULI

There is a wealth of information in the fundus of the eye for any physician with an ophthalmoscope. Practice looking at the fundus of young persons, such as your classmates. Young people have bigger pupils, more patience, and usually no opacities of the cornea, lens, or vitreous. The retina in a young person is glistening and shiny with beautiful sharp details.

The first time you examine a retina, it is probably best if you and the subject are standing. You have more mobility and will be less awkward. However, as soon as you know how to do it, and as a regular practice, always sit and have the patient sit. Do not sit directly in front of the patient so that your knees hit his; sit facing him with your chair to one side of his. When you get to be an expert, you can examine supine patients, but do not do it until you have to.

- Ask the patient at the start not to hold his breath. This has a practical application on the size and pulsations of his retinal veins.

• With the patient sitting with his back to the window, pull the blinds down and ask the patient to remove his glasses. You do not need a blacked-out room, but remove any incidental light.

There are two things working against you when you use the ophthalmoscope. First, the eye adds all the light it is exposed to. The sum of the ambient light and the ophthalmoscope light, plus the balance between sympathetic and parasympathetic tone, plus the fact that the pupillary sphincter muscle is stronger than the dilator, determines the pupil size. Second, trying to look through a *reflecting* surface is difficult. On a sunny day you cannot look into a lake to any depth because of the reflection off the surface. However, if you hold a hat close to the water and look into the lake in the shadow of the hat, you can see into the water. Similarly, side light or ceiling light reflected on the patient's cornea or surface of his glasses will hinder you. When you examine the patient's fundus, you will partially eliminate reflections by holding the ophthalmoscope so close to the patient that it is touching her forehead. If you rotate the ophthalmoscope 5 or 10 degrees while holding it vertically, the light from the scope strikes the cornea at different angles and you will find the best "reflection-free" angle.

Some doctors keep their glasses on when using the ophthalmoscope; most, however, remove them.

1. **Unless you have marked astigmatism, take your glasses off.** With your glasses off, the head of the ophthalmoscope can be closer to your eye and you will see a larger area of the patient's retina. Try it both ways, beginning with your glasses off. The pinhole effect (see under "Near Vision") of looking through the viewing aperture (Figure 1–1) may take care of your refractive error. If you are astigmatic, your glasses contain a cylinder; hold your glasses at arm's length, look through one lens with one eye and slowly rotate your glasses to the right and then to the left. If the object you are looking at tilts and elongates at one point in the rotation, then your prescription includes a cylinder; you are astigmatic, and you may have to wear your glasses when using the ophthalmoscope.

2. **Hold the ophthalmoscope in your right hand, turn it on, and look through the viewing aperture. You must get the viewing aperture as close as possible to your eye.** The soft rubber bar (Figure 1–1) horizontally placed across the top of the ophthalmoscope head is meant to fit firmly against or just below your eyebrow. There should be some contact between your skin and the rubber bar at all times when you are looking at the fundus oculi. Keep your index finger on the lens selector wheel. If you have the ophthalmoscope halfway down your nose, you

are, in effect, looking through a tube with your pupil at one end and the viewing aperture at the other.

3. **Use your right eye to examine the patient's right eye and vice versa.** However, if you have one "weak" eye, use the other for examining both of the patient's eyes.

4. **Hold the ophthalmoscope in your right hand when examining the patient's right eye and in your left hand when examining the patient's left eye.**

5. **Keep the ophthalmoscope vertical, and keep both your eyes open.**

6. **When examining the patient's right eye, put your left hand on top of the patient's head (Figure 1–2B) and rest your forehead on your flexed thumb and vice versa when examining the left eye.** Ask the patient to stare at something at eye level on the other side of the room and to keep her eyes as still as she can. To examine the patient's right fundus, stand to the patient's right (not directly in front of her) about 60 cm from her. With the ophthalmoscope head up against your eye, shine the light in her right and left eyes by rotating the vertically held ophthalmoscope (Figure 1–2A). You will see two red-orange circles, the red reflexes (much like the reflections of a car's headlights in a cat's eyes at night); these are the patient's retinas.

Follow down onto the right red circle by moving closer to the patient (Figure 1–2C). If you lose the red reflex, move back and start over. Adjust the

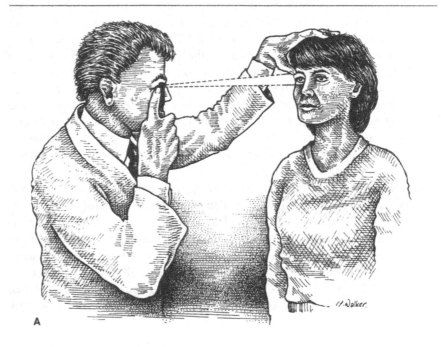

A

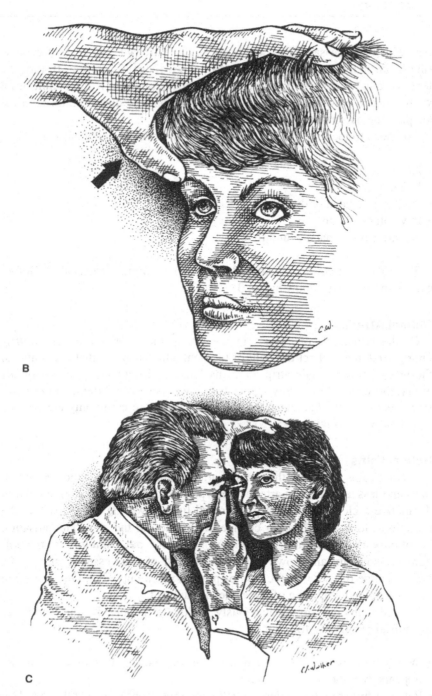

B

C

Figure 1–2. A. Examining the right retina. Stand in front and to the right of the patient. The red reflex, which is the reflection off the retina, is easily seen although the examiner is 60 cm from the patient. The examiner's forehead will rest on his left thumb. **B.** The examiner's left hand and flexed thumb (arrow) provide a pivot for his forehead. **C.** The final position puts the examiner as close as possible to the patient.

lens wheel if necessary. This will bring any fine artery at the edge of the disc (the head of the optic nerve) into clear, sharp focus. Starting at 0, turn the lens selector wheel one or two clicks in either direction. If the definition of what you see is worse, turn the wheel in the opposite direction, all the time keeping the ophthalmoscope up to your eye.

You need to identify the following and know normal from abnormal:

- Arteries
- Veins
- Optic nerve head or disc
- Physiological cup
- Posterior pole, macula, and fovea

The following comments are helpful when examining each other. Before examining patients, read Chapter 3.

Retinal Arteries

Of the two kinds of vessels in the retina, the arteries are the *smaller*. Orange-red, they reflect the light of the ophthalmoscope so that the center of the artery shows a pale strip along its length. The thicker the wall of the artery, the wider is the shiny white strip down its center. Arteries do *not* pulsate and are somewhat angular. They cross and more commonly are crossed by retinal veins (Figure 1–3).

Retinal Veins

Retinal veins are larger than retinal arteries and are a dusky red. More sinuous and less angular than arteries, they pulsate. Retinal veins do not have as distinctive a clear white strip of reflected light down the center. To see the pulsations, look for a bend or change in direction of the vein. The pulsation is not only an expansion of the caliber of the vein, but a *shunting* of the column of blood up and down within the length of the vessel (Figure 1–4). Veins change direction at the disc or physiological cup edge. One can often see a filling and emptying of the vessel at the bend.

Retinal veins pulsate spontaneously in 80% of people. If you cannot see the pulsations, try the following:

- Watch the biggest vein you can see at the edge of the disc or where it disappears over the edge of the cup.
- Put your finger on the patient's eyelid and press gently against the eye. You will see the vessels empty as the intraocular pressure rises.
- If you let go suddenly, the venous pulsations often become visible.

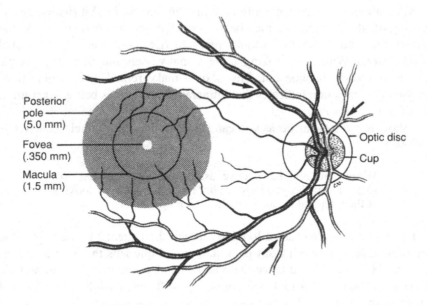

Figure 1–3. Details of the retina. The posterior pole and the macula are not this well-defined in the living retina. The branching vessels (arrows) indicate the direction to the disc.

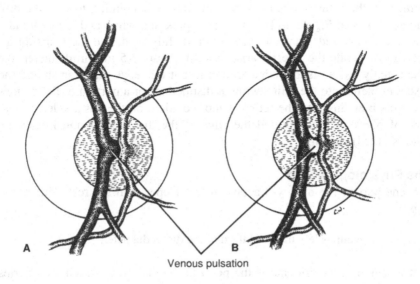

Figure 1–4. A. Retinal vein pulsation at the point where the vein disappears into the physiological cup. The vein is filled. **B.** As in A, but with the vein empty.

Alternatively, ask the patient to take in a big breath, hold it (which means closing off the glottis), and then bear down (the Valsalva maneuver). As the intracranial and intraocular venous pressure rises, you can see the retinal veins distend. While still looking at the retinal vessels and after 30 s, ask the patient to slowly breathe out. This should make retinal venous pulsations visible. The pulsation indicates that intracranial pressure is below 200 mm of water *at that moment.*

Follow the vessels as far as you can peripherally. You can help yourself as follows:

> When examining her left eye, ask the patient to turn her eyes
> to her left while you move to her right; you are now looking
> at the temporal periphery of her left retina.

This is not easy. Instead of looking through the patient's round pupil, you are now looking through a slit pupil and an oblique lens that induces astigmatism. However, if you brace the ophthalmoscope against yourself and the patient and ask her to look left, right, up, and down while you look and move in the opposite directions—and persist at it—you will be able to see the peripheral retina.

The Head of the Optic Nerve or Disc

The disc is located at the nasal side of the center of the retina. The V formed by the bifurcations of veins and arteries is pointing toward the disc (small arrows in Figure 1–3). The disc is pink and white and is much paler than the orange-red retina. It is round or slightly oval, and the veins disappear into it while the arteries arise from it. About 1.5 mm in diameter, the disc usually has a distinct edge around it, but this edge may vanish and the disc will blend into the retina without distinction for a portion of the periphery. This blending into the retina is more evident on the nasal side. A crescent of black pigment around the edge of the disc is common in myopic (shortsighted) persons.

The Physiological Cup

Some part of the disc will appear to be deeper than the rest. This is the cup.

> The cup is less than one third of the disc's diameter.

It is usually eccentric and is the point in the disc from which the arteries arise and the veins enter. There may be pearly white fibers, the lamina cribrosa, making a crosshatched appearance on the floor of the cup. It is important for you to learn the size of the physiological cup relative to the disc and the depth of the cup in those with normal vision (see the section on "Glaucoma" in Chapter 2).

The Posterior Pole

The central region of the retina is divided clinically and anatomically into three areas. The clinical and anatomical terminologies are not the same. In this manual *clinical* terminology is used. The anatomical equivalents are given in parentheses.

We have to consider the following:

• Posterior pole (macula or area centralis)
• Macula (fovea)
• Fovea (foveola)

The **posterior pole** is about 5 mm in diameter. Its outer limits cannot be clearly defined clinically. Histologically, it has more than one layer of ganglion cell nuclei.

The **macula** is at the center of the posterior pole and is a shallow depression about the same size as the disc. It is a darker red than the rest of the fundus, opposite the center of the pupil, and you will not see it well without dilating the pupil. Never give your opinion on its appearance without first dilating the pupil.

• You can see the macula by asking the patient to look into the ophthalmoscope light.
• Look at the retina. You will see several small groups of arteries coming off the temporal side of the disc that rapidly curve toward each other in a vertical direction. They end by surrounding the macula (Figure 1–3).

The **fovea** is the center of the macula. A depression seen as a yellow-white reflecting spot, it lies two disc diameters to the temporal edge of the disc, about 1 mm below its center.

Keep the following points in mind when using the ophthalmoscope:

• Examine the fundus of the eye with the patient sitting.
• Keep the patient's back to the window, with the overhead lights out.
• Ask the patient not to hold his breath.
• Hold the ophthalmoscope vertically.
• It is easier for the patient if you decrease the intensity of the ophthalmoscope light when looking at the posterior pole.

- Keep your right eye opposite the patient's right eye, and keep both your eyes open.
- Do not breathe into the patient's face.

If the patient wears glasses, ask him to take them off. Look at them. If they are *plus* lenses, as you look through them and move them from side to side, objects move in the *opposite* direction. The reverse is true for the myope who wears minus lenses. For the myope you need a negative (red-numbered) lens in the ophthalmoscope to see retinal details clearly. Start with 0 showing at the lens strength window, and with your finger changing the lens wheel in the opposite direction of the arrow (counterclockwise) (Figure 1–1), you will soon see a clearly defined retina.

You do not need to do anything to allow for a patient with astigmatism, although many astigmatics are also myopic. For a hyperopic patient, reverse the procedure described for a myope. Start with 0 at the lens strength window, but turn the lens selector in the direction of the arrow (clockwise).

When you become proficient at using the ophthalmoscope, you may leave the patient's glasses on and look through them; this is especially helpful in **high myopia**. However, there are disadvantages: (a) both the inside and outside surfaces of his lens reflect incidental light and (b) his glasses prevent you from getting close to his eye and thus reduce the area of his retina that you can see.

Finally, do not spend too long on this part of the examination; you cannot see all there is to see in each patient until you have looked in several hundred eyes. Get to know each feature of the retina individually by looking in every eye that you can, irrespective of the patient's complaints.

VISION

The following terms should be familiar to you:

Amblyopia: Reduced visual acuity

Aphakia: Absence of the lens, such as following cataract removal or dislocation of the lens out of the pupil area

Astigmatism: Impairment of eyesight usually caused by unequal curvature of the cornea

Hypermetropia: Same as hyperopia

Hyperopia: Farsightedness, or focusing of light behind the retina

Myopia: Nearsightedness, or short sight; light focuses in front of the retina

Presbyopia: Impairment of eyesight because of old age

Vision is discussed here in two parts—**central**, or **macular**, **vision** and **peripheral vision**. Central vision can be measured as both near and distance vision.

Central Vision

Distance Vision

Always test and examine the right eye first.

Measure distance vision by using a test card of letters of different sizes. Distance vision is expressed as visual acuity (VA). This is a test of macular function. In the examining room use a Snellen card placed 6 m from the patient. There are also cards for use at 3 m from the patient (Figure 1–5A). The card should be well lit.

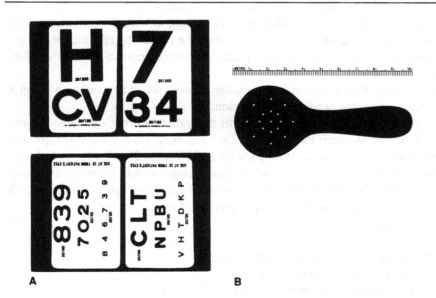

A   B

Figure 1–5. A. Plastic 6 × 9–cm cards for measuring visual acuity at 3 m. **B.** Plastic pinhole for verifying a refractive error.

Ask the patient to put on her glasses, cover one eye, and read the letters or numbers (or E chart for those who are illiterate) downward, that is, from the bigger to the smaller characters.

The smallest line of readable symbols is the patient's VA, which is expressed as a fraction. The numerator is the distance in feet or meters at which the test is made, and the denominator indicates the distance at which someone with normal vision would be able to read the line. If the patient can read the 20-ft (or 6-m) line when the card is 20 ft (or 6 m) away, her vision is 20/20 (or 6/6) and she has normal macular function. Less than normal ranges from 20/25 to 20/400.

If the patient can read all the letters except one in the 40-ft line, her vision is recorded as 20/40-1. Similarly, if she can read all the letters except two in the 60-ft line, her vision is 20/60-2. If she misses more than two letters in any line, her visual acuity is that of the next line up.

If the patient cannot see the largest letter, hold your hand about 1 m in front of the eye being tested and, with three or four fingers outstretched, ask her, "How many fingers can you see?" If she answers correctly, record this as CF (counting fingers) at 1 m.

Lesser vision than this should be tested and recorded as HM (hand movements) only at 1 m, and even lesser vision should be tested by directing a bright light into one eye from 0.3 m—recorded as LP (light perception) only. A finding of no light perception indicates a sightless eye.

There are Snellen test cards to be used at 6 m, or with the card on the wall above and behind the patient's head, while the patient faces a mirror at 3 m. Distance vision can be recorded from 6/60 to 6/6 (normal) and better than normal as 6/4.

For the patient who has forgotten his glasses, see the remarks on using a pinhole, under the heading "Near Vision."

Test visual acuity in each eye with the patient's other eye covered *and* with both eyes open. Patients with cataracts may have VA 20/60 right and left when the eyes are tested separately and 20/30 to 20/40 when tested with both eyes open. Also, patients with latent nystagmus may have normal acuity with both eyes open. When one eye is covered, the nystagmus occurs in both eyes and the acuity decreases in the uncovered eye.

Remember:

- Visual acuity is a test of macular function.
- Visual acuity is expressed as a fraction.
- The numerator is the distance at which the test is made.
- The denominator is the distance that a person with normal vision can read

the smallest line readable by the patient.
- Measure the best corrected vision of each eye separately, right then left, and both together.

Near Vision   The patient with cataracts may have quite good distance vision and poor near vision, and the myope can read newsprint without his glasses but has poor distance vision. Near vision can be tested using the print in a telephone directory or a newspaper. Formal testing requires Jaeger's test type or Birmingham Optical Group test card or the American Medical Association test card. The patient holds the card in his hand at a comfortable distance and reads the smallest typed paragraph that he can. Glasses must be worn; test each eye separately, then together.

If the patient has forgotten his glasses, a pinhole will help (Figure 1–5B). If the patient holds the pinhole up to his eye and reads the test card through one of the holes, refractive errors are eliminated. The light coming through the pinhole is axial and remains unrefracted by the patient's cornea and lens and is sharply focused on the macula.

Whether the person is myopic, hyperopic, or presbyopic, testing his vision with the use of a pinhole will bring his vision up to normal. If it does not, his loss of vision is not a result of refractive error.

Figure 1–5A is a reproduction of two pocket cards used to test visual acuity. They are lettered and numbered and are used at 3 m. Similar cards are available at most surgical supply houses or medical college bookstores. Get a set and put them in your ophthalmoscope case with the pinhole.

Peripheral Vision

Peripheral fields of vision reflect the function of the retina (the nonmacular part) and the visual pathways connected to the nonmacular retina. When testing *acuity*, letters and parts of letters and numbers of different size that subtend a portion of an arc are used. When testing *peripheral fields*, the stimulus is movement.

To test visual fields by **confrontation**, seat the patient facing you with his glasses off. Ask him to cover his right eye with his hand and to stare at your right eye with his left eye. Hold your arms out to either side so that your fingers are at the *edges* of his visual fields, as in Figure 1–6A. If the examiner has his right hand at A in Figure 6A, he will get no responses from the patient, as the test object (his moving finger) is behind the patient's field and the patient cannot see it, let alone say whether or not it is moving. If the examiner's right hand is at B, then the test object is inside the field, not on the edge, and a substantial crescent of blindness could be present in the patient's left temporal field and yet be missed because the test is being done incor-

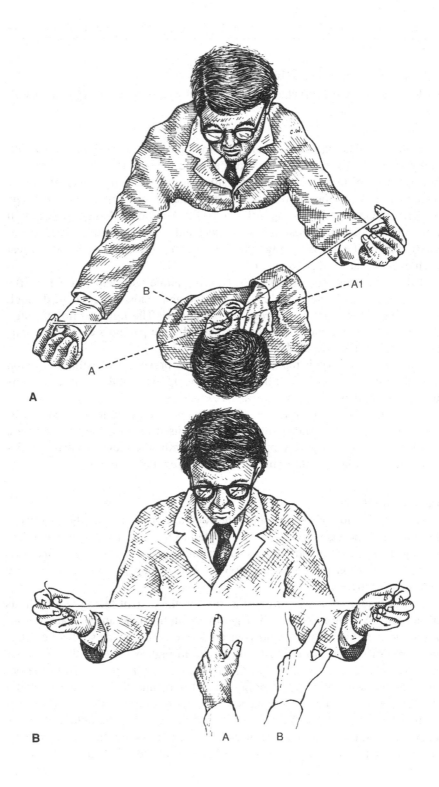

A

B

rectly. Keep the examining fingers on the *edges* of the fields. Start with your hands behind the patient's vision at A and A1. Bring your hands forward, one at a time, while wiggling your fingers until the patient can see them. You have thus discovered the edges of the fields and are ready to start testing.

It is important to have the patient continue staring at your right eye with his left. Ask him to tell you on which side he sees fingers moving, that is, right, left, or both. Some patients cannot or will not say "right" or "left." They sometimes mean their right and sometimes your right, and doctor and patient can both become confused. You may ask the patient to *point* to the side that moves and say "both" if both move. Alter the moving side randomly, sometimes right, sometimes left, and sometimes both. Test in both the upper and lower portions of the visual fields.

> Do not test with your fingers on the equatorial line of the fields or on the midsagittal meridian.

With a test object as big as your moving finger, you will not know whether you are in the upper or lower half of the field. These halves are anatomically distinct. Test the upper halves well up in the field and the lower halves well down in the field. If movement in any area is being ignored, move the hand toward the midline until it is seen to be moving. Keep the movement small, that is, only a *portion* of one finger, and *slow*. Coarse, fast movements are much easier to see than fine, slow ones.

> Always move both right and left fingers simultaneously at least twice in the upper portion of the fields and again in the lower portion.

Simultaneous right and left stimulation is valuable. A patient may be able to see all the movements along the left edge and all the movements along the right edge when the two sides are examined individually. However, when the two sides are stimulated *simultaneously*, the competitive effect of the two *simultaneous stimuli* may bring out a consistent visual field defect. This kind of field defect is not an absolute defect, but is known as an **inattention field defect**.

← ─────────────────────────────────────

Figure 1–6. A. Testing the field of vision of the patient's left eye by confrontation. Points A and A1 are behind the edges of the field, point B is well inside the field, and the examiner's fingers are correctly placed on the *edges* of the field. **B.** Visual field assessment of the patient who cannot or will not fix. Ask him to quickly point to the center of the string. If his hand is at A, his lateral fields are approximately full; if at B, he has a left hemianopia (see text for using the string test).

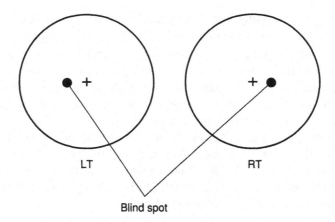

LT   RT

Blind spot

Figure 1–7. Record the patient's visual fields with his right eye field on your right. Mark his right field with *Rt.* and his left field with *Lt.* Indicate central vision with a plus sign. Add the visual acuity (corrected or uncorrected), date, and shade the blind areas.

Sometimes you cannot get the patient's cooperation, and field testing by confrontation will not work. Try the string test as shown in Figure 1–6B. Hold a piece of string with your hands about 24 in apart. Without a lot of instruction or warning, ask the patient to *quickly* point to the center of the string. If his fields are full (from side to side), he will point to the approximate center. If he has a field defect on his left, he will point to the right of center. This can be used to detect altitudinal defects as well if you hold the string vertically.

Finally, in uncooperative patients whose disease is clearly in the hemisphere(s), it is often impossible to test one eye alone. Such patients cannot or will not keep one eye closed. Therefore, you may have to examine the fields with both eyes open, and if the lesion is retrochiasmal, this is good enough.

Visual fields may also be tested by perimeter. This creates a permanent record of visual field loss.

A Bjerrum's screen is used for the formal examination of the central, as opposed to the peripheral, visual fields.

When making notes about visual fields, draw the patterns in the patient's history as though they were your own fields (Figure 1–7), that is, the right eye field on your right and the left eye field on your left. Include the visual acuity and date.

Although visual fields are not really round and they overlap on the nasal side, they are usually drawn this way. The plus sign in the center represents

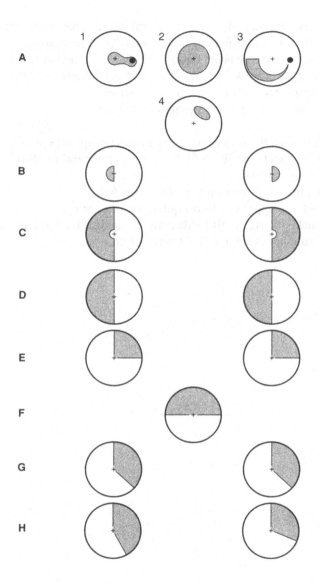

Figure 1–8. Various field defects. **A.** Scotomas: 1—cecocentral, 2—central, 3—arcuate, 4—paracentral. **B.** Bitemporal central scotomas. **C.** Bitemporal complete hemianopia with sparing of central vision. **D.** Left complete homonymous hemianopia with splitting of central vision. **E.** Right upper quadrantanopia. **F.** Altitudinal or horizontal field defect (upper). **G.** Incomplete congruous right homonymous hemianopia. **H.** Incomplete asymmetrical congruous right homonymous hemianopia.

central vision. The shaded oval area, lateral to the center and partially astride the equatorial line, is the normal blind spot. This is an absolute scotoma representing the optic nerve head, or disc, which has no retinal function.

You need to be familiar with the types of field defects shown in Figure 1–8 and their significance. (The blind areas are shaded.)

In testing visual fields by confrontation, remember:

- The patient must fix his gaze on your eye and keep this eye still.
- No one can detect color or definition in his peripheral fields of vision—the stimulus is movement.
- Keep your testing fingers on the *edge* of his fields.
- Test in both the upper and lower quadrants of each eye.
- Always make the right half fields compete against the left half fields by offering simultaneous right and left stimulation.

Loss of Vision 2

This chapter includes a list of definitions you need to know, a few anatomical hints about the visual system, and a listing of some of the kinds of visual problems you can expect to encounter.

Listed with each disease are some common or typical characteristics that will help you with recognition. Some of these diseases do not "belong" in the neurologist's examining room, but you cannot preselect your patients. Although the neurologist's opinion is often not the final word on a problem of visual loss, you must know how the visual system works and how diseases of this system present themselves.

DEFINITIONS

Visual acuity: Literally, visual "sharpness" tested by evaluating the recognition of patterns of letters or numbers, graded sizes, brightness discrimination, and color recognition

Macular vision: Same as central vision, the zone in the center of the **field of vision**. It extends as a circle from fixation about 15 degrees. Visual acuity is a measurement of the integrity of macular vision.

Peripheral field of vision: All of the area of space that can be seen, exclusive of central vision, when the eye is stationary. The extent of the peripheral field is (from fixation) about 60 degrees on the nasal side and upward, about 70 degrees inferiorly, and about 90 degrees on the temporal side. The nasal fields of the two eyes overlap.

Scotoma: An area of decreased or absent vision *surrounded* by an area of normal vision. A scotoma may be relative or absolute. A scotoma is *relative* if a small test object cannot be seen in it but a sufficiently large object can be seen. It is *absolute* if nothing can be seen in it.

Central scotoma: A scotoma that includes the fixation point; visual acuity is decreased. The bigger it is, the larger will be the letter on the Snellen test type that may be "hidden" in the scotoma and the worse will be the visual acuity (type 2 in Figure 1–8A).

Cecocentral scotoma: A horizontal oval scotoma including fixation and extending to and including the blind spot (type 1 in Figure 1–8A)

Arcuate scotoma: As seen in type 3 in Figure 1–8A, corresponds to and represents nerve fiber bundle loss

Blind spot, or physiological scotoma: The area of blindness in the field of vision resulting from the head of the optic nerve. It is oval, 5 degrees wide and 8 degrees high, and on and mostly below the equator on the temporal side of fixation. Its nasal side is about 12 degrees from fixation. It cannot be seen with both eyes open because of the visual field overlap.

Find your own blind spot. Close your left eye. Stare at something at eye level straight ahead of you with your right eye (do not move your eye!). Hold a pencil in your right hand at arm's length. Move the pencil in from the temporal side, on the equator or just below it. As your pencil approaches fixation, you will find you can "lose" the eraser on the end of the pencil in your blind spot. You can slide the eraser around in the blind spot. This is how central field defects are plotted. If you cannot find it, you are not *fixing* your right eye on a distant object.

Hemianopia: Loss of half of the field of vision in both eyes or either eye

Homonymous hemianopia: Loss of half of the field of vision in each eye and on the *same* side of the midsagittal meridian in each eye; that is, a left homonymous hemianopia means the patient has lost vision in his temporal half field of the left eye and nasal half field of the right eye. A bitemporal or binasal field defect may be hemianopic but it is not homonymous. Loss of vision in the upper or lower field respecting the equator and ignoring the midline vertical meridian is called an altitudinal defect (upper or lower) and may be congruous or incongruous (discussed later in this chapter; see also Figures 1–8H and 2–5).

Bitemporal hemianopic central scotoma: The scotomas are in the temporal halves of macular vision. The nasal sides are intact and acuity is normal. The peripheral field is normal (Figure 1–8B). (a) Hemianopia with *splitting* of the macula—the vision in *half* the peripheral field and *half* the macula is gone, but visual acuity is normal (Figure 1–8D). (b) Hemianopia with *sparing* of the macula—the vision in half the peripheral field is gone, but all of macular or central vision is normal and, of course, acuity is normal (Figures 1–8C and 2–7). (c) Hemianopia with macular loss—hemianopia as above plus all of macular vision and *abnormal* visual acuity. This is not a hemianopia plus a central scotoma. By definition, a scotoma is an area of blindness surrounded by normal vision.

The visual cortex is all of Brodmann's areas 17–19. Area 17 is the primary visual cortex receiving the optic radiation from the lateral geniculate body.

Area 17 is the striate cortex, area 18 is the parastriate cortex, and area 19 is the peristriate cortex.

The striate cortex is striated by a light strip of myelinated fibers parallel to the surface of the cortex and known as Gennari's line. You can see it easily with the naked eye in a fresh brain.

Seven important points about the visual pathways are:

1. Optic inversion: Everything you can see from the right eye is divided in two ways. There is a vertical meridian dividing it into the right (or temporal) field and the left (or nasal) field. Everything in the *temporal* field is perceived by the *nasal* retina, and vice versa for the nasal field.

Also, there is an equatorial division. Everything below it is perceived by the upper retina, and vice versa for things above it.

In addition, the nerve fibers in the visual pathways arising from both temporal retinas do *not* cross the midline and they end in the ipsilateral occipital cortices. All the fibers arising from both nasal retinas *do* cross the midline and thus end in the contralateral occipital cortices.

On the medial surface of the occipital lobe you can see the calcarine sulcus, which is roughly horizontal and divides the occipital lobe into upper and lower portions.

All the nerve fibers arising from cells in the retinas above the horizontal division end up in the occipital cortex above the calcarine sulcus and below it for the fibers originating below the horizontal.

The retina is well organized, like a pie divided into four more or less equal pieces, plus the central plum for the posterior pole. In contrast, the visual *fields* are not equal. The temporal field is 60–70% bigger than the nasal field, yet each has about the same amount of retina. Each of the four retinal "pieces" is anatomically distinct with its own connections. The occipital cortex is clearly divided by the calcarine fissure in the horizontal plane. However, the arrangement of fibers in the visual pathways between the retina and the occiput is not so methodical. For example, macular fibers in the optic nerve immediately behind the eye are in the upper lateral part of the nerve. Immediately in front of the chiasma the same fibers are in the center of the nerve. The chiasma, optic tract, lateral geniculate body (LGB), and optic radiation each have their unique fiber arrangements and proportions of fibers or cells (LGB) devoted to peripheral or central vision. [There is an excellent picture of this on page 916 of the 35th edition of *Gray's Anatomy* (Warwich and Williams, editors), Longman, 1973.]

As an example of proportion, the posterior pole of the retina is about 5 mm in diameter and the macula is about 1.5 mm. The whole retina, when laid out flat, is about 50–55 mm across; thus, over 90% of the retina is devoted to peripheral vision. By contrast, in the occipital cortex the amount of brain representing central vision is huge relative to the amount concerned with the peripheral fields. The occipital cortex representing central vision is the *most posterior* part of the occipital pole, and the peripheral retina is represented by the most anterior part of the occipital cortex.

In general, upper retinal fibers remain upper and lower ones remain lower except in the optic tract and the LGB, where a 90-degree rotation occurs. The rotation becomes undone in the optic radiation.

2. Lesions of the retina and optic nerve are characterized by unilateral, central, altitudinal, ring, and cecocentral scotomas; diminished visual acuity; altered color vision; and afferent pupillary defects. The opposite eye remains normal.

3. Chiasmal lesions are characterized by bitemporal defects. They may be in the peripheral field, the central field, or both (Figure 1–8B and C). Progressive lesions posterior to the chiasma will eventually cause homonymous field defects. The chiasma is about 1 cm above the pituitary gland. This large space can accommodate relatively large suprasellar tumors with no field defect. Although the chiasma is directly above the dorsum sella in most patients, it may be located more anteriorly or posteriorly. This variability will account for atypical field defects. There are unique fiber arrangements in the chiasma.

   a. **Ventral nasal optic nerve fibers** (serving the superior temporal field) cross in the anterior chiasma and loop into the distal opposite optic nerve and then turn posteriorly to the contralateral optic tract (see Figure 2–1).

   b. **Macular fibers** make up a large part of the chiasma and are located largely inferiorly.

   c. **Nasal macular fibers** decussate in the posterior chiasma. (Figures 2–1 to 2–4 are applicable to chiasmal lesions.)

4. Optic tract lesions are characterized by their incongruity. They usually begin as a quadrantic defect with early sparing of macular vision (Figure 2–5).
5. Optic radiation:
   a. In *temporal* lobe lesions, field defects are principally superior and quadrantic; if hemianopic, they are denser and earlier in the *upper* quadrant.
   b. In *parietal* lobe lesions, field defects may be inferior and quadrantic but, more commonly, hemianopic. When early and progressive, they will be denser and first evident in the *lower* quadrants (Figure 2–7).
6. Occipital lobe: Monocular temporal crescent, field, or scotomatous defect, in *anterior* occipital lobe lesions (Figures 2–9 and 2–10).
   a. Central, congruous scotomas, in lesions of the *tip* of the occipital pole (Figure 2–8).
   b. Hemianopic with macular sparing; bilateral lesions will leave the patient with tubular vision, that is, all blind but for 10 degrees around fixation, or all central and peripheral loss.
7. The more posterior the lesion, the more likely are the areas of field defect in the two eyes to be congruous and macular vision spared. Macular fibers in tract, LGB, and anterior optic radiation are confined to a relatively narrow area. Posteriorly, they form a large part of the radiation and cortex.
8. Visual field defects are congruous when they are the same *shape* in each eye and incongruous when they are not. Unless they are hemianopic, they are seldom the same *size*. Optic radiation lesions are commonly congruous, and tract lesions are usually incongruous.

DIAGNOSIS

The location of the lesion is often obvious in visual system disease because of the *pattern* of the area of visual loss; for example, when visual acuity in the right eye is reduced to 20/200 with a central scotoma but the left eye is normal, the lesion must be between the right cornea and the optic chiasma. When the visual acuity is normal and there is a right upper homonymous quadrantanopia (Figure 1–8E), the lesion must be in the left temporal lobe involving the optic radiations.

As a generalization, the findings of central (type 2 in Figure 1–8A), ring, arcuate (type 3 in Figure 1–8A), or cecocentral (type 1 in Figure 1–8A) scotomas, visual loss in one eye only, abnormal color vision, and afferent pupil defect (see Chapter 5), or an altitudinal field loss (Figure 1–8F) are indicative of disease in the retina or optic nerve.

Normal visual acuity with field defects on the same side of the vertical meridian (ie, homonymous) are caused by lesions in the optic tract, LGB, optic radiation, or occipital cortex. The more posterior the lesion, the more likely the field defect in one eye will be congruous with the defect in the other eye (Figure 1–8G). If the field defect is a *complete* homonymous hemianopia, you cannot tell where the lesion is, except that it must be behind the chiasma.

More diagnoses are missed because of a failure to appreciate the arrangement of the fibers in the optic chiasma than any other part of the visual system.

Histories vary from helpful to misleading. The presbyopic patient complains he cannot get far enough from his newspaper to read it. (The ability to read the fine print in the average newspaper requires 20/30 vision.) The patient with pigmentary retinal degeneration will often forget to mention the progressing night blindness, an extremely important symptom. Another patient with an *inattention* left hemianopia has no complaints and is being examined only at the insistence of, for example, his wife or the motor vehicle licensing authorities. Typically, in the past months he has been driving with the left side of his car over the dividing line into oncoming traffic.

The patient who says he covered one eye with his hand and realized he was virtually blind in the other eye has told you nothing about the tempo of the disease, but has revealed that the lesion is between his cornea and the chiasma.

Also, some people are born with one eye myopic and the other eye normal and they discover the fact incidentally. A man of 40 who wears no glasses and has no visual complaints gets a foreign body in his eye (not in the line of vision). When the foreign body is successfully removed, he discovers that the vision in the previously injured eye is not as good as in the other eye. In his mind the injury and the diminished visual acuity are cause and effect. Examination shows reduced visual acuity but an otherwise normal eye. The pinhole improves his visual acuity to the 20/20 line. Refraction by an ophthalmologist confirms that his best corrected vision is normal. This eye has always been myopic and the trauma has simply brought it to his attention.

When confronted with an apparent recent loss of vision in one eye that makes no sense, *always* get a full refraction before conducting more elaborate investigations.

SOME DISEASES OF THE VISUAL SYSTEM

Retina and Optic Nerve Lesions

Retrobulbar Neuritis Retrobulbar neuritis typically presents in young adults, with onset over 24–48 hr, a large central scotoma, and a painful eye on palpation and movement. There may be a past history of episodes of multiple sclerosis or this illness may be the first manifestation of it. The fundus is usually normal. Afferent pupillary defect is commonly present.

Optic Neuritis   The presentation of optic neuritis is like that of retrobulbar neuritis, except that it may be painless. The terms *retrobulbar neuritis* and *optic neuritis* are used interchangeably. Edema of the optic nerve head may be present. (See the section on papillitis in Chapter 3.)

Central Serous Retinitis   Central serous retinitis has subacute onset (days) of slight to moderate vision loss in one eye, usually in a male patient aged 20–40. The disease is caused by fluid exudate lifting the retina, usually at the macula. The patient complains that objects look smaller with the affected eye.

Giant Cell Arteritis of the Central Retinal Artery   This disease occurs in those age 60 or older, with a sudden onset of central blindness. Superficial temporal arteries are typically tender, pulseless, and tortuous. There is almost always an elevated erythrocyte sedimentation rate and a low-grade fever. The history will often contain complaints of headache and stiff, aching, weak shoulder and hip muscles. Funduscopy shows total retinal ischemia (see the following section). Diagnosis, including temporal artery biopsy, is an emergency.

Anterior Ischemic Optic Neuropathy   In patients over age 50, anterior ischemic optic neuropathy is a manifestation of giant cell arteritis, vasculitis, diabetes mellitus, or Takayasu's disease or is frequently idiopathic. There is a sudden onset of visual loss, sometimes followed by increasing and progressive visual failure over 5–7 days. Altitudinal (inferior) field defects are common. Funduscopy examination shows a swollen disc, hemorrhages near the disc edge, and cotton-wool spots. A macular star is common with vasculopathies. The other eye is commonly involved within weeks or months of the first eye.

Retinitis Pigmentosa   The most common symptom of retinitis pigmentosa (RP) is night blindness. The onset and severity of symptoms depend on the pattern of inheritance: the autosomal recessive type presents earliest and is the most severe, X-linked is intermediate, and autosomal dominant is frequently mild. The fundus shows black "bone spicules" of pigment clustered around vessels in the midperiphery. The disc is waxy pale, and there is attenuation of both retinal vessels. Visual fields show ring-shaped arcuate or annular scotomas.

Pseudoretinitis Pigmentosa Pseudoretinitis pigmentosa refers to the fundus findings of a number of disorders that mimic RP. Some pigmentary retinopathies that are *not* RP are those following congenital and acquired syphilis, childhood exanthemas, phenothiazine usage, and trauma.

Atypical RP includes sectoral RP (fundus changes in one sector of the fundus bilaterally, which can mimic chiasmal lesions) and pericentral RP (fundus changes central). Unilateral RP probably does not exist.

Diseases and syndromes associated with RP are Bassen-Kornzweig, Bardet-Biedl, Kearns-Sayre, and Usher's.

Glaucoma Glaucoma exists when elevation of **intraocular pressure** is sufficient to damage optic nerve fibers at the optic disc level. This is the second leading cause of blindness in North America. There are two types: acute angle-closure glaucoma (ACG) and chronic open-angle glaucoma (OAG).

ACG presents with severe pain in the eye and head, blurred vision, and colored halos around lights, plus nausea and vomiting. Pain results from a rapid rise in intraocular pressure. Attacks are precipitated by reduced illumination and may be relieved by sleep, bright light, or miotic agents, all of which constrict the pupil. ACG usually presents unilaterally. The predisposing factors are often bilateral, and the uninvolved eye is therefore at risk. **This is an emergency.**

OAG is the most common form of glaucoma and is **dangerous** because the onset is often gradual and asymptomatic. Central vision is preserved until late, and the field loss is often unnoticed by the patient until the disease is well advanced. It is usually a bilateral disease, although asymmetrical.

Visual field defects in glaucoma respect the *horizontal* division of the visual fields. The arcuate nerve fibers arching above and below the macula from the temporal region are most susceptible to glaucomatous damage. Therefore, the characteristic field defects are paracentral and arcuate nasal scotomas (type 3 in Figure 1–8A). The central area of the visual field is the most resistant, so visual acuity may be normal even in advanced glaucoma.

Optic disc changes are an increase in the *diameter* and *depth* of the physiological cup and increased pallor.

Central Retinal Vein Occlusion Central retinal vein occlusion (CRVO) presents with painless, always unilateral, loss of vision. The patient is commonly a young adult. The extent of visual loss is variable, depending on the degree of venous occlusion, the amount of macular edema, and the presence or absence of complications such as retinal neovascularization and neovascular glaucoma.

The fundus shows dilated, tortuous veins; retinal hemorrhages usually in the peripheral retina; and retinal edema. Cotton-wool exudates are usually seen only around the disc. The disc edge is indistinct, although the physiological cup remains visible.

Visual fields reveal a relative central scotoma and acuity is usually 20/100, improving to 20/60 with time if there are no complications.

Branch retinal vein occlusion is most common in the superotemporal branch. Fundus changes are confined to the distribution of the branch, and field loss is segmental.

Hypertension often coexists with CRVO, and associated retinal artery disease is a common finding. A picture similar to that of CRVO may be seen in hyperviscosity syndromes, leukemia, and myeloma.

Retinal Artery Occlusion   Retinal artery occlusion (RAO) is accompanied by sudden, painless, unilateral loss of vision. It is commonly discovered by the patient on awakening in the morning and occurs in the stroke-prone age group. If the central retinal artery is involved, vision will be completely lost (no light perception). If a cilioretinal artery is present, an island of central vision will be preserved. Visual loss may be confined to a segment of the field if only a branch of the retinal artery is occluded.

The fundus reveals a gray, opaque, edematous retina with a cherry-red fovea. This is normal choroid contrasted against gray retina. Splinter hemorrhages are rarely seen. Branch arteries may show segmented columns of blood (boxcars). There may be a history of transient monocular visual loss lasting minutes, with altitudinal progression as vision fails, that is, the window blind effect.

Causes of RAO include emboli, thrombosis, giant cell arteritis, and collagenvascular diseases.

Retinal Detachment   Retinal detachment (RD) presents with a history of recurrent flashes or floaters in the same area of the visual field. The patient typically complains of a cloud or curtain obscuring part of the field. It usually starts and is most dense peripherally and extends toward central vision. Visual acuity is normal unless or until the macula detaches. An inferior detachment with a superior field defect can be present for a long time before the patient is aware of it. The fundus shows an elevated retina that is gray and wrinkled and undulates.

The elevation will be appreciated as you rack in progressively more plus lenses (black numbers) on the ophthalmoscope to keep the elevated retina in focus.

The most common predisposing factor to RD is degenerative retinal change (as seen in high myopia). Other causes include trauma; a simple "black eye" history may be significant. Malignant melanoma of the choroid can cause a secondary RD, and the retinal neovascularization of diabetes mellitus may result in a tractional RD.

Macular Degeneration Macular degeneration begins at any age but is most common over 60 years. Slow loss of visual acuity occurs bilaterally and is worse in bright light and better in the dark; recovery of vision is slow after exposure to a bright flash of light. The macula may appear normal initially. There are central and paracentral scotomas. Fluorescein retinal angiography and the Amsler grid are helpful in diagnosis.

Optic Neuropathy Optic neuropathy can occur:

1. Without other diseases (eg, Leber's). The typical patient is a young adult male with loss of central vision in one eye, followed by the other eye in days or weeks, with a positive family history. Characteristic fundus changes in the acute stage are followed by optic atrophy. A central scotoma will become cecocentral with upper nasal breakout.
2. With other central nervous system (CNS) diseases, with one or more of the following: congenital deafness, ataxia, spastic quadriparesis, mental deterioration, polyneuropathy, Friedreich's ataxia, Marie's cerebellar ataxia, and Charcot-Marie-Tooth disease
3. With inborn lysosomal disorders: (a) mucopolysaccharidoses or (b) lipidoses

Optic Atrophy Optic atrophy occurs as a consequence of the foregoing and other diseases, such as methyl alcohol or chloroquine ingestion, isoniazid toxicity, and any compressive, ischemic, or toxic disorder of the retinal ganglion cell or fiber from the retina to the LGB. This includes papilledema, which, if severe enough or chronic enough, can result in optic atrophy. Diagnosis of the cause is often impossible. Clinical diagnosis of atrophy is dependent on the color and structure of the disc.

The lesion responsible for optic atrophy may be anywhere from the retina to the LGB inclusive.

Chiasmal Lesions The most common visual field defect is bitemporal, either central or peripheral or both.

Be careful and persistent with patients with visual loss. Lesions in the chiasmal region can be deceptive and extremely chronic. The chronicity and slow progression seem to make the symptoms more acceptable and less demanding. Every neurologist and neurosurgeon has had some bad experience with patients thought to have multiple sclerosis, amblyopia from childhood, low-tension glaucoma, retinitis pigmentosa sine pigmento, or atypical macular degeneration as an explanation for their blindness who eventually turn out to have a chiasmal lesion as the true cause. It does not help the patient to make the diagnosis after the optic atrophy is marked and the acuity is down to 20/200.

Another reminder about chiasmal lesions is the place of exploratory intracranial surgery. Ordinarily, there is no such operation as an exploratory intracranial procedure. However, if an eye and field examination point to a chiasmal lesion, even if the skull x-ray, carotid angiography, computerized tomography (CT) scan, and nuclear magnetic resonance (NMR) studies are all normal, then the next "investigative" step is **exploration of the chiasmal area**. The neurosurgeon may make the diagnosis of chiasmal arachnoiditis that cannot be treated, but he may find the otherwise undiagnosable 4-mm meningioma, pituitary tumor, or craniopharyngioma.

Finally, lesions of the visual pathways behind the optic chiasma never interfere with color vision (ie, without an accompanying loss of light perception). There are reported examples of defective color appreciation from a parietal cortical lesion, but this is color agnosia, not loss of color vision.

Anterior Chiasmal Syndromes

1. The ipsilateral eye is blind and there is an upper temporal field defect in the contralateral eye. The lesion is shown at **a** in Figure 2–1A.

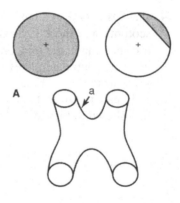

Figure 2–1A

2. The ipsilateral eye is blind and there is a central temporal scotoma in the contralateral eye (The same lesion as in Figure 2–1A).

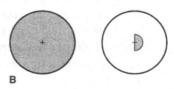

Figure 2–1B

3. The ipsilateral eye is normal and the contralateral eye is as in Figure 2–1A or B (The same lesion as in Figure 2–1A).

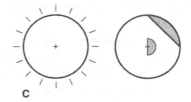

Figure 2–1C

4. The ipsilateral eye has a central scotoma and there is a paracentral scotoma in the temporal field of the contralateral eye (The same lesion as in Figure 2–1A). This can progress to the condition shown in Figure 2–1E.

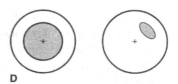

Figure 2–1D

5. The ipsilateral eye is blind and there is a paracentral scotoma in the temporal field and full peripheral field of the contralateral eye (The same lesion as in Figure 2–1A).

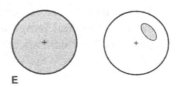

Figure 2–1E

Chiasmal Body Bitemporal peripheral field loss occurs as in Figure 2–2A or central temporal scotomas occur as in Figure 2–2C, or a combination of the two as in Figure 2–2B. Lesions occur as in Figure 2–2D. The lesion is usually below the chiasma (eg, a pituitary tumor).

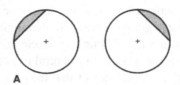

Figure 2–2A

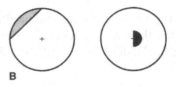

Figure 2–2B

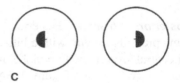

Figure 2–2C

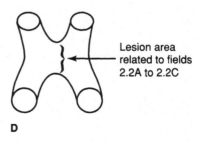

Figure 2–2D

Suprasellar lesions (eg, cranio-pharyngioma, aneurysm, meningioma, chordoma, or third ventricle disten-tion) can start with a central or periph-eral temporal defect that initially may be most marked inferiorly as in Figure 2–2E.

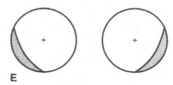

Figure 2–2E

Any of these lesions (suprasellar or infrasellar) may eventually produce the field defect shown in Figure 2–2F.

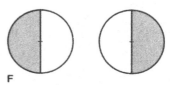

Figure 2–2F

Posterior Chiasma Posterior chi-asma presents usually with a bitempo-ral central scotoma with peripheral de-fects as well, as in Figure 2–3A. A central scotoma usually occurs first. The lesion is shown at **a** in Figure 2–3B. When big enough to involve the tract at **b,** a homonymous, hemianopic defect is added.

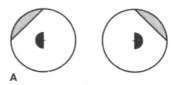

Figure 2–3A

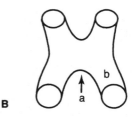

Figure 2–3B

Lateral Chiasma Lateral chiasmal lesions present with nasal field defects. Very rare, they can be unilateral as in Figure 2–4A or bilateral as in Figure 2–4B. The defect rarely comes up to the midline. Unilateral nasal defects have been reported as a result of infarction of the optic nerve, aneurysm, pituitary tumor, and ectatic carotid artery. Bilateral nasal defects have been reported resulting from chiasmal arachnoiditis and secondary to obstructive hydrocephalus and pressure from above from the third ventricle. **Glaucoma** is probably the most common cause of nasal field defects.

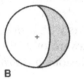
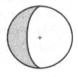

A

Figure 2–4A

B

Figure 2–4B

Optic Tract Lesions

Optic tract lesions between the chiasma and the LGB produce incongruous field defects as in Figure 2–5.

Most lesions behind the chiasma, whether tract, LGB, radiation, or cortex, present as homonymous field defects with normal visual acuity. The lesions cause loss of vision in some or all of the two homonymous half fields. When the hemianopia is *complete*, the site of the lesions cannot be located by visual field examination alone.

Blind areas resulting from tract lesions are homonymous and extremely incongruous in shape and size.

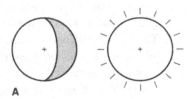

Figure 2–5

1. When a tract lesion produces a complete hemianopia, the eye contralateral to the lesions will show an afferent pupil defect (see Chapter 5). This may be difficult to elicit.
2. When a tract lesion presents with some degree of hemianopic visual loss *plus* decreased visual acuity and color vision, the lesion has involved the chiasma or the optic nerve(s). This area is compact, and distances are small.
3. Some lesions originate in or near the sella and then expand laterally to involve the tract. The patient may present with the confusing combination of a chiasmal (bitemporal) defect plus an optic tract (incongruous hemianopic) defect.
4. Many patients with lesions *anterior* to the LGB (ie, tract, chiasmal, and nerve) are aware of a dimness or loss of vision. Conversely, most patients with lesions *posterior* to the LGB are unaware of their visual defect.

Optic Radiation

Within the Temporal Lobe A homonymous defect, superior and quadrantic, is shown in Figure 2–6.

Defects can be congruous or incongruous. When incongruous, the larger defect is usually in the eye on the *same* side as the lesion. It is also denser in this eye. The blind area may cross the horizontal division of the visual fields.

When the defect is incongruous, it is never as incongruous as with optic tract lesions.

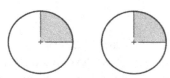

Figure 2–6

Within the Parietal Lobe A hemianopic homonymous defect may initially be *only*, or denser, in the lower fields, as in Figure 2–7.

This is congruous with sparing of the central vision and normal acuity.

Peripheral defects result from medially placed lesions.

There is an abnormal optokinetic response (see Chapter 6).

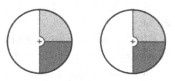

Figure 2–7

Occipital Lobe and Visual Cortex Lesions

The more posterior the homonymous defect, the more likely it is to be completely congruous.

Tip of occipital pole lesions can produce central homonymous scotomas with precise congruity. Figure 2–8 shows a field defect recorded by Sir Gordon Holmes. The tip of the patient's right occipital lobe was injured with the resulting left incomplete homonymous hemianopic central scotomas.

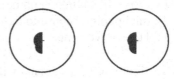

Figure 2–8

Anterior Visual Cortex or Posterior Optic Radiation

There are *unpaired* nasal fibers that correspond to the extreme temporal peripheral field and the most anterior aspect of the area striata. In patients with posterior optic radiation lesions, there may be a unilateral **temporal crescent defect** as in Figure 2–9. It may be above or below the horizontal division and often is the forerunner of a hemianopic defect. The defect may be a temporal crescent scotoma *not* touching the edge of the field (not shown). Thus, a postchiasmal lesion may produce a purely monocular field abnormality.

The *sparing* of a thin temporal crescent of vision when the rest of the temporal field is hemianopic also occurs as in Figure 2–10.

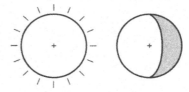

Figure 2–9

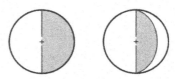

Figure 2–10

Cortical Blindness

The term *cortical blindness* is used synonymously with *bilateral homonymous hemianopia*. The definition includes

* Loss of all vision, including perception of light
* Loss of reflex blinking on being threatened
* Normal pupil response to light and convergence
* Full eye movements

It is common for patients with this disorder not to complain of the vision loss or to deny the blindness when confronted with the fact (Anton's syndrome). Remember that the condition commonly occurs from occlusion of the upper end of the basilar and the two posterior cerebral arteries. As the latter supply the inferior and medial surface of the temporal lobes as well as the primary visual cortex, an acute confusional amnesic syndrome may accompany the acute loss of vision. The latter may account for the denial of the blindness; that is, it is an agnosia.

The Abnormal Retina

3

PAPILLEDEMA

Terms synonymous with *papilledema* which are in common use are *choked disc*, *swollen disc*, and *swelling of the nerve head*.

Definition

Papilledema is a swelling (laterally) and an elevation (anteriorly) of the disc. It is caused by increased intracranial pressure and is measured in diopters. (A diopter is a unit of refraction; that is, a lens with a power of 1 diopter has its principal focus at a distance of 1 m.) Only the elevation and swelling of the disc are papilledema.

Restrict the term *papilledema* to nerve head swelling caused by increased intracranial pressure. Other causes of swelling and elevation of the nerve head should be named from the causative process, for example, optic neuritis, anterior ischemic optic neuropathy, or hemorrhagic retinopathy.

The characteristics of *early papilledema* include the following:

1. **Disc hyperemia** results from dilatation of capillaries on the surface of the disc.
2. The retina immediately *surrounding* the disc becomes dull, loses its linear light reflexes, and is a dusky red. The disc margins blur.
3. Venous pulsations—which disappear late in fully developed papilledema—are *not* a useful *early* sign. The level of increased intracranial pressure varies, and when it drops below 200 mm of water, the veins then pulsate. Also, not all people with normal intracranial pressure have pulsatile retinal veins.
4. Venous dilatation and tortuousity is not in itself a good early sign.
5. Nerve fiber hemorrhages—thin radial streaks on the disc or near its edge—are a highly reliable confirming sign.
6. Nerve head elevation is the sine qua non of papilledema (see below).

In *fully developed papilledema* the following occurs:

1. Engorged, tortuous, dusky retinal veins are present, the disc is elevated and margins of the disc are unidentifiable, and there is marked capillary

dilatation over the disc. In addition, there are many flame-shaped and splinter hemorrhages in the retina and (if the pressure increase has been rapid) globular subhyaloid hemorrhages. In advanced papilledema you will also see cotton-wool spots, macular exudates forming an incomplete stellate pattern around the macula, and retinal wrinkling (Paton's lines).

2. In chronic papilledema the disc elevation remains, the hemorrhages and exudates resolve, and nerve fiber loss may be seen. The end state is optic atrophy.

How to See It

- When examining patients, start with a plus 8 (black number); you see an orange blur.
- Turn the lens selector wheel counterclockwise using progressively weaker plus lenses until the surface of the disc is sharply defined. Note the magnification (eg, +4).
- Look at the patient's fundus again *beside* the disc and keep decreasing the plus lens until retinal details come into focus (eg, +1).

The difference in these two readings is the amount of papilledema in diopters, that is, 3. (We cannot use a lens of less than 1 diopter. A difference between the nerve head and surrounding retina of less than 1 diopter is too subjective to be meaningful.)

About 3 diopters are equal to 1 mm of change. The target to be seen clearly is usually the smallest vessel you can see. You do not need a patient with papilledema to learn this; one of your classmates has a normal physiological cup. You can see the bottom of it with great clarity using a (for example) −2 (red number) in your ophthalmoscope. He has a fine artery in the retina to one side of the disc. You will see this vessel with great clarity by using a +1 (black number), that is, 3 diopters, or three clicks on the scope; the retinal vessel is about 1 mm closer to you than the bottom of the cup.

Remember, the higher the plus lens you use, the shorter the focal length and the more anterior is the part of the patient's eye you can clearly see, for example, with a +20 lens in the window of the ophthalmoscope you will focus on his cornea. The more negative the lens, the longer the length and the farther back in the patient's eye is the point of focus; for example, −50 to −10 enables you to focus on the retina of the myopic patient with the long oval eye.

> Do not look at the fundus with a zero lens in the ophthalmoscope and plan to increase the plus lenses as you concentrate

on the elevated disc, thinking it will become clear while the surrounding retinal details blur. Your own accommodation will not allow it, and you will miss the papilledema.

Remember:

1. Start plus (eg, +8); aim the light at the disc.
2. Diminish the lens strength (by a counterclockwise turn on the lens selector wheel).
3. Stop when the disc is clearly seen.
4. Note the lens number.
5. Aim *beside the disc* at the retina.
6. Diminish the lens strength.
7. Stop when retinal details are clearly seen.
8. Note the lens number (the difference is the amount of papilledema).

The normal eye is shown in cross-section in Figure 3–1A, and the disc area is shown in more detail in Figure 3–1B. The disc is 1.5 mm in diameter and, seen with the ophthalmoscope, looks like those in Figures 1–3 and 1–4.

The disc edges are of different elevations at various points on the circumference of the nerve head. The physiological cup is a true depression in the nerve head. There is no retina overlying the nerve head, hence the normal blind spot.

The optic nerve is surrounded by a sheath space continuous with the subarachnoid space surrounding the brain (Figure 3–1B). This space, which contains spinal fluid, may be filled with blood, inflammatory products, or spinal fluid under increased pressure in various disease states.

Figure 3–2A and B shows cross-sections of a papilledematous eye. The nerve is swollen, bulging forward, and expanded. Notice in Figure 3–2B how the retina is pushed *laterally* by the bulging nerve head.

Examine both eyes, because the amount of papilledema is frequently different in the two eyes. Look in both eyes and judge them independently.

Visual Acuity

Uncomplicated papilledema of moderate duration and degree does not interfere with visual acuity. Clearly, acute papilledema with a hemorrhage into the macular area will diminish visual acuity.

Severe and long-standing papilledema can produce optic atrophy and blindness. In the chronically compressed optic nerve both glial cells and small vessels proliferate, and if the swelling is severe, necrosis of the nerve may occur.

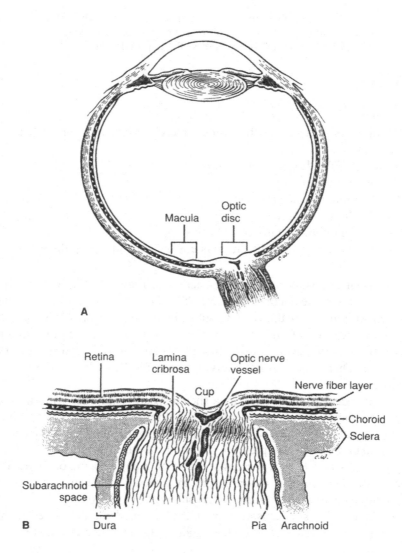

Figure 3–1. A. Cross-section of the normal eye. The optic disc is on the nasal side of the macula, which is in the posterior pole of the eye. **B.** Profile of the optic nerve, disc, cup, and subarachnoid space surrounding the nerve.

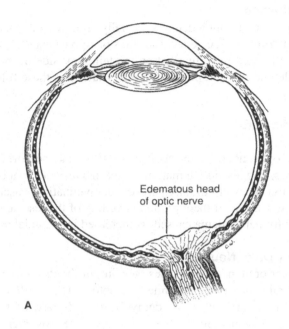

Edematous head
of optic nerve

A

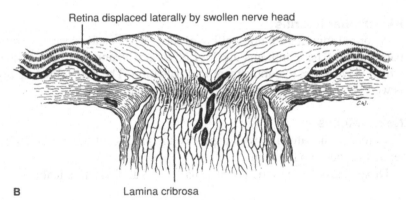

Retina displaced laterally by swollen nerve head

B   Lamina cribrosa

Figure 3–2. A. Cross-section of the eye with papilledema. The nerve head is expanded forward and, as seen in more detail in B, spreads *laterally*, displacing the
retina. **B.** The edematous optic nerve head is expanded forward and laterally. The
retina is displaced and wrinkled.

Retinal Wrinkling

In the presence of papilledema (especially chronic), one can see wrinkling of the retina. You will see concentric folds or ripples parallel and close to the edge of the disc and most marked on the temporal side of the disc. As long as the swollen nerve head pushes the retina laterally, these folds will persist.

OTHER DISEASES

Papillitis, optic neuritis, retrobulbar neuritis, and neuroretinitis, by their word endings, suggest inflammation of the nerve head (papillitis) or nerve trunk (neuritis). They are usually part of a demyelinating, vascular, or inflammatory process. Some of them produce swelling of the disc, and therefore can be mistaken for papilledema caused by increased intracranial pressure.

Papillitis, or Optic Neuritis

Papillitis, or optic neuritis, causes swelling of the disc of about 2 diopters. Loss of central vision is the prominent symptom. There will also be evidence of a vascular, inflammatory, or demyelinating disease of the optic nerve head. There may be pain in the eye at rest or on eye movement *only*.

Retrobulbar Neuritis

A normal fundus with no swelling of the disc is usually seen with retrobulbar neuritis. The symptoms are loss of central vision and pain in the eye, which is worse on eye movement and palpation. The demyelinating process is well behind the eye, hence the term *retrobulbar*.

Neuroretinitis

Similar to the situation with papillitis, the process of neuroretinitis has extended farther into the retina.

These diseases (eg, optic neuritis) have several distinctive features:

1. Loss of vision—This may be a central or paracentral scotoma or a huge island of blindness involving the whole or almost the whole field of vision (in contrast, in early papilledema an enlarged blind spot is usually the only vision change).
2. Pain on eye movement (or on palpation of the eye and sometimes at rest)—This is presumably a result of traction and swelling of pain-sensitive structures at the apex of the orbit. The pain is more common with retrobulbar neuritis than with papillitis and may be present or absent with either. The pain usually precedes the blindness by 1–2 days (in contrast, papilledema is painless).

Hypertension

There are several systems for grading the fundus changes in hypertension (eg, grade I or grade II). Do *not* do this: describe what you see. Hypertension produces a number of changes and signs in the fundus:

1. Diffuse and focal or segmental constriction of the retinal arteries—The older the patient, the less significant is the arterial narrowing. The earliest narrowing occurs in the retinal periphery. Tortuousity of the arteries is most evident at the disc edge, and this change is indistinguishable from arteriosclerotic changes unrelated to hypertension.
2. Disc edema—It looks the same as disc edema resulting from any other cause.
3. Arteriovenous "nicking"—This may produce relative venous obstruction and retinal hemorrhages distal to the arteriovenous crossings.
4. Retinal hemorrhages—Widely distributed over the retina (in contrast, a radial arrangement is seen around the disc in papilledema), petechial and larger and often round, as well as flame-shaped. Look distal to the arteriovenous crossings.
5. Exudates (spots, streaks, and clusters of white to gray material in the retina)—These may be arranged radially around the macula in a star configuration.

Remember:

1. Increased intracranial pressure may produce papilledema.
2. Start with a +8 to +10 lens, diminishing the magnification until the disc is in focus. Note the magnification and then diminish the magnification further until the retina is in focus.
3. The more acute the onset of the papilledema, the more hemorrhages are present; these are arranged radially around the disc.
4. Vision is initially normal, with an enlarged blind spot.
5. Papillitis and retrobulbar neuritis may cause nerve head swelling; characteristically, these cause central blindness and eye pain.
6. Elevated blood pressure may cause disc edema:
   a. With diffuse and focal arterial changes
   b. With venous nicking and venous obstruction at the arteriovenous crossings
   c. With a variety of hemorrhages diffusely seen in the retina often from veins distal to the arteriovenous crossings
   d. With exudates

Eye Movements, Diplopia, and Cranial Nerves 3, 4, and 6

4

DIPLOPIA

When a patient says he has double vision, his eyes are no longer in alignment. He has a disease of the third, fourth, or sixth cranial nerve or a disease of one of the six muscles that move the eye, or of the myoneural junctions.

You can make yourself have double vision. Do this and you will understand better what the patient is talking about. Keep both your eyes open. Put your left index finger horizontally on your left upper eyelid. Do not cover the pupil. Gently press the left eye down. Hold your pen horizontally at arm's length in your right hand. Look at the pen as you move it toward the floor. You see two pens, one above the other. The farther downward you move the pen, the greater is the separation between the two images. They are parallel, one above the other. If you close your right eye, the top pen (the true image, the macular image, the sharp one) disappears. If you close your left eye, the bottom pen (the false image, the fuzzy one) disappears.

Double vision results from light reflected off an object and onto the macula of one eye (the nonparalyzed one) and onto the retina, near the macula, of the other eye. The true image is the macular one, and the false image, which is always less distinct, is the nonmacular one. The greater the nonalignment of the paralyzed eye, the greater is the separation between the two images. When a patient says she is seeing double and her right eye is turned in toward her nose, she has a weak right lateral rectus. If her right eye is turned down and out and she has a drooping right upper eyelid and an enlarged pupil, the patient has a third nerve lesion on the right. Usually, however, the eyes seem to move in a normal way. Therefore, a system of examining eye movements is necessary.

Definitions

Abduction: Movement of the eye in the horizontal plane *away* from the midline

Adduction: Same as for abduction but *toward* the midline

Cover test: Have the patient fix on the Snellen chart at his line of best vision. Cover one eye. If the other eye moves to take up fixation, a tropia exists. The movement will be seen in the uncovered eye irrespective of which eye is covered. On the other hand, if a covered eye moves to fixate when uncovered, a phoria exists. The other uncovered eye does not move.

Depression: Same as for elevation but *downward*

Elevation: Movement of the eye in the vertical plane *upward*

Esophoria: A deviation of the eye *toward* the other eye when the stimulus of vision has been removed

Esotropia: A *manifest* deviation of the visual axis of one eye *toward* the other; also known as convergent or internal strabismus, or cross-eye

Exotropia: A *manifest* deviation of the visual axis of one eye *away* from that of the other; also known as divergent or external strabismus, or walleye

Heterophoria (latent strabismus): Failure of the eyes to remain parallel after the stimulus for binocular single vision has been removed (by covering one eye, as in the cover test). A phoria may be inadvertently demonstrated in the course of retinal examination when the head and ophthalmoscope of the examiner interfere with the patient's fixation and the eye being examined turns as the examiner withdraws.

Hypertropia: A deviation of the visual axis upward

Hypotropia: A deviation of the visual axis downward

Rotation (as you face the patient): *Inward,* or *internal*—Rotation of the eye so that the 12-o'clock point on the cornea turns toward the nose, that is, clockwise rotation of the right eye, counterclockwise rotation of the left eye. *Outward,* or *external*—Rotation so that the 12-o'clock point turns away from the nose, that is, counterclockwise rotation of the right eye, clockwise rotation of the left eye

Squint: In North America this word sometimes means to screw up the facial muscles around the eyes as though looking into a bright light. In medicine, it means to have an external eye muscle palsy or a permanent **strabismus.**

Strabismus: A deviation of the eye that the patient cannot overcome

The other heterophorias are *hypophoria*, in which the visual axis of one eye sinks below the other; *hyperphoria*, in which the visual axis of one eye rises above the other; and *cyclophoria*.

See the section on "Paralytic Versus Concomitant (Nonparalytic) Strabismus."

How to Discover the Muscles Responsible for Double Vision

- Test the function of the third, fourth, and sixth cranial nerves together.
- Have the patient seated, facing you.
- Put your left hand on top of the patient's head so it will not move when he is moving his eyes from side to side.

We test *saccadic* movements (command) by asking the patient to look right, left, up, and down and *pursuit* movements by having him follow an object. Test both. Some diseases affect one type of movement but not the other.

1. **Hold a pen 0.5 m in front of the patient's nose.** If your pen is any closer, you are making his eyes converge at the same time the other movements are being examined.
2. **When examining lateral eye movements, hold the pen vertically; when testing up-and-down movements, hold the pen horizontally.** If you test lateral eye movements by holding the pen horizontally, the patient will have to separate the two images by the *length* of the pen in order to see two pens. If you hold the test pen vertically, he will need only to separate the two images by the *width* of the pen in order to see two.
3. **Move your pen from side to side, asking the patient to follow it with his eyes.** The area of lateral *binocular* vision is limited by the bridge of the nose and how far the eyes are sunk into the head. From Figure 4–1 it is clear that double vision can occur only when an object is between C and B. There cannot be binocular double vision lateral to C or B.
4. **Test the vertical movements once with the patient's eyes turned to the right halfway between looking straight ahead and an extreme right lateral gaze, and once with the eyes to the left, halfway between looking straight ahead and an extreme left lateral gaze.**

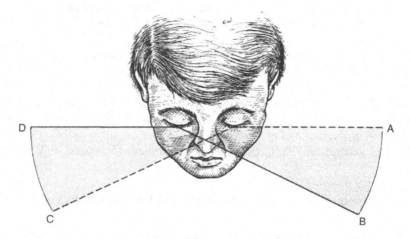

Figure 4–1. The range of binocular vision is between C and B. Objects between C and D can be seen with the right eye only, and those between A and B are visible with the left eye only.

5. **Test the lateral movements to the right and left with the eyes starting in the primary position.** Stay in the binocular field (Figure 4–1).

Rule 1

> In the analysis of any diplopia, put the eyes in the position that causes the greatest separation of the two images.

For example, let us assume that the separation is greatest on looking up and to the left.

Rule 2

> Discover from which eye the false image is coming.

The false image is the nonmacular, less distinct, image. It is always the outside image; that is, if the diplopia is lateral with two images side by side, the image farther away from the midline is the false one. If the diplopia is vertical with two images one on top of the other and maximum separation occurs when the patient looks up, the false image is the one closer to the ceiling. With a vertical diplopia and maximum separation when looking down, the false image is closer to the floor. This is true whether the ocular palsy is divergent or convergent.

> The next step is to cover either eye. Ask the patient which image disappears. Give him several chances while you slowly cover and uncover one of his eyes and he holds his gaze so that the two images are maximally separated. If he tells you the near or inside image always disappears when you cover his right eye, then the outside image must vanish when you cover his left eye. The false image is coming from the left eye, and the left eye is thus the paretic one.

Rule 3

> Determine what muscle moves the eye in this particular direction and what is the nerve supply of that muscle.

Maximal separation is up and to the left, and the false image is from the left eye. The elevator of the left eye when the eye is abducted is the superior rectus, the nerve supply of which is the third cranial nerve. Therefore, the cause of diplopia is a partial left third nerve palsy.

FUNCTIONS OF THE EXTERNAL OCULAR MUSCLES

Six muscles move each eye, and none of them has a *single* function. Each has a major and a minor function. The six muscles are the four recti (medial, lateral, superior, and inferior) and the two obliques (inferior and superior). *Rectus* means "straight."

Lateral Rectus

Primary Function The lateral rectus muscle is supplied by the sixth cranial nerve (the **abducens**).

1. Its primary function is abduction, the most common extraocular paresis you will encounter.
2. Head posture is important. With paresis of the *left* lateral rectus, the chin is turned toward the left shoulder as the patient faces you. The eyes are thus out of the area of control of the left lateral rectus.
3. Images are side by side; the outside image, farther from the patient's nose (the paralytic, or false, image), disappears when the left eye is covered. Conversely, the inside image disappears when the right eye is covered.

4. The diplopia will be greatest at a distance and lesser for near vision if weakness of either lateral rectus muscle is the cause of the diplopia.

Secondary Function   The lateral rectus muscle has a slight but definite **inhibition of vertical eye movements,** both up and down.

In a left lateral rectus palsy, when the patient looks to the left there are two images, the most lateral from the left eye, the most medial from the right eye. When she looks to the left and up, the most lateral image is from the left eye but there is now vertical separation of the two images and the *top* one is from the *right* eye.

If she looks down and to the left, the image from the left eye is most lateral but the *bottom* one is from the *right* eye. The logical conclusion from this mess is (a) a left lateral rectus palsy (correct) and (b) a right superior and inferior oblique muscle palsy (wrong).

When the left lateral rectus is paralyzed, the **inhibition of elevation and depression** is lost as well as the *abductor* function. Therefore, the eye has increased mobility upward and downward when it moves to the left as far as the weak lateral rectus will take it. This overly mobile up-and-down movement of the left eye may be misinterpreted as *reduced* mobility, up and down, of the adducted right eye.

A comparable secondary function with vertical separation exists for paresis of the **medial rectus** (see below).

To summarize, the lateral rectus is a primary abductor and secondarily inhibits elevation and depression of the abducted eye.

Medial Rectus

The medial rectus muscle is supplied by the third cranial nerve (the oculomotor).

1. Its primary function is *adduction.*
2. Its secondary function is to inhibit elevation and depression of the adducted eye as the lateral rectus does of the abducted eye.
3. When the *right* medial rectus is paretic, the patient will sit facing you with his chin toward his *left* shoulder and his right eye *abducted.*
4. With the images side by side, the greatest separation occurs when the patient looks to the left. The outside image will vanish when you cover the right eye.

Superior Rectus

The superior rectus (one of two eye elevator muscles) cannot do its principal job of elevation with the eye in the primary position because the long axis of the muscle is not parallel to the anteroposterior axis of the eye (Figure 4–2A).

1. The superior rectus is supplied by the third cranial nerve. Fibers arising from the *right* oculomotor nucleus supply the *left* superior rectus and vice versa. It is a pure *elevator* of the eye, only when the eye is *abducted* as in Figure 4–2B.
2. When the right eye is adducted as in Figure 4–2C, the superior rectus acts as an inward rotator—its secondary function.
3. In all other positions it has mixed functions, elevation and rotation.
4. When the superior rectus is paretic, the patient's chin is up, with the head extended and tilted toward the shoulder of the opposite side.
5. When the two images are positioned one above the other (you may have to hold up the patient's ptotic eyelid with your finger), maximum separation (for right superior rectus weakness) is up and to the right. The top image is from the right eye.

Inferior Rectus

The inferior rectus is one of the two eye depressor muscles.

1. It is supplied by the third cranial nerve.
2. The primary function is as a *depressor* when the eye is *abducted.*
3. Its secondary function is as an *outward rotator* when the eye is adducted (opposite to the superior rectus).
4. When the right inferior rectus is paretic, the patient's chin is down, the image separation is greatest when the gaze is down and to the right, and the false image is closer to the floor.

Superior Oblique

The superior oblique is one of the two eye depressor muscles.

1. It is supplied by the fourth cranial nerve (the trochlear). *An anatomical reminder:* The fourth cranial nerve is the only cranial nerve coming off the dorsum of the brain stem. Also, the nerves decussate before they emerge, so the left trochlear nerve supplies the right superior oblique muscle and vice versa. The oblique muscle rises in the apex of the orbit and its tendon runs through the pulley (trochlear) and then runs posterolaterally to insert in the posterior part of the eye behind the equator (Figure 4–3A and B).
2. Its primary function is *depression* of the *adducted* eye.
3. Its secondary function is inward rotation of the abducted eye.

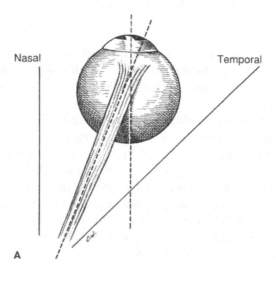

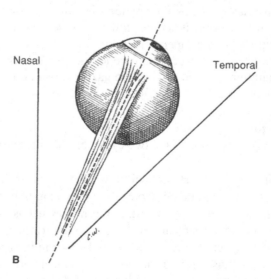

Figure 4–2. The right eye from above, showing the superior rectus muscle. **A.** The eye is in the primary position. The long axes (dashed lines) of the eye and the superior rectus muscle are not parallel. **B.** With the eye abducted, the axes are parallel and the superior rectus muscle is an elevator. (*Continued*)

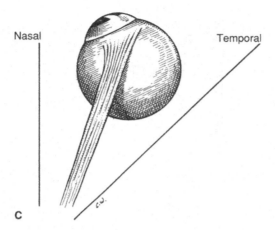

Figure 4–2 (continued). C. With the eye adducted, the superior rectus muscle is an inward rotator.

4. When the right superior oblique is paretic, the patient's chin is down and her head is tilted and turned with the left ear to the left shoulder (not reliable).
5. Image separation is greatest when the patient is looking down with the right eye adducted. One image is above the other; the false image is lower, tilted, and coming from the right eye.

Inferior Oblique

The inferior oblique is one of the two eye elevator muscles.

1. It is supplied by the third cranial nerve.
2. Its primary function is *elevation* of the *adducted* eye.
3. Its secondary function is outward rotation of the abducted eye.
4. When the right inferior oblique is paretic, image separation is greatest when the patient looks up with the right eye adducted. The false image comes from the right eye, is tilted, and is above the true image.

Tertiary Functions

1. The superior and inferior recti are *adductors* and assist the medial rectus, becoming more effective as adduction increases (see above for

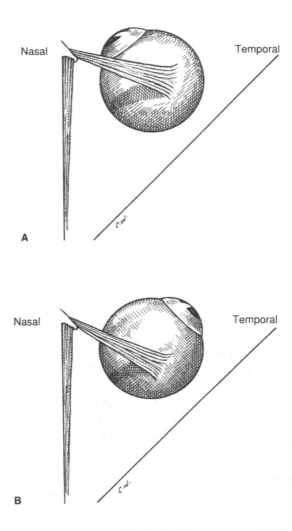

Figure 4–3. A. The right eye from above. The superior oblique muscle acts as a depressor when the eye is adducted. **B.** The superior oblique muscle acts as an inward rotator when the eye is abducted.

comments regarding the superior rectus not being straight unless the eye is abducted). This tertiary function is nil when the eye is abducted.

2. The superior and inferior obliques assist the lateral rectus and are *abductors* of the already abducted eye. Their abducting function is nil when the eye is adducted.

Summary

- When the eye is *abducted*, the superior rectus elevates, the inferior rectus depresses, and the obliques rotate.
- When the eye is *adducted*, the superior oblique depresses and the inferior oblique elevates, while the superior and inferior recti rotate.
- The two elevators are the superior rectus and the inferior oblique.
- The two depressors are the inferior rectus and the superior oblique.
- The *superior* rectus and *superior* oblique are inward rotators ("SIN" may be used as a memory jogger).
- The *inferior* rectus and *inferior* oblique are outward rotators.
- The superior and inferior recti add to adduction; the two obliques add to abduction.
- The lateral and medial recti inhibit elevation and depression.
- When an extraocular muscle is paralyzed, have the patient fix with the paretic eye alone and the normal eye alone. The deviation (of the normal eye) is always *greater* when the paretic eye is fixating and less (of the paretic eye) when the normal eye is fixating.

WHEN TO EXAMINE FOR ROTATION

If both elevator muscles and both depressor muscles are working, you cannot see rotation, as the rotatory effects of the superior rectus and superior oblique (inward) and the inferior rectus and inferior oblique (outward) balance each other.

In a third nerve palsy the unopposed lateral rectus muscle abducts the eye. The medial rectus is paretic and cannot adduct. The superior oblique will not depress the abducted eye. The only movement left to test on the superior oblique is its rotary function, as both outward rotators (inferior oblique and inferior rectus) are paretic and cannot oppose the inward rotation of the superior oblique. Do the following:

- Pick out a scleral conjuctival vessel on the temporal side and another on the nasal side of the globe and watch them.
- Ask the patient to look *down* and *out*; the movement will not be marked.
- If the fourth cranial nerve and superior oblique muscle are working, the temporal vessel moves up and the nasal vessel moves down (ie, inward rotation).

PARALYTIC STRABISMUS VERSUS CONCOMITANT (NONPARALYTIC) STRABISMUS

Concomitant Strabismus

A **concomitant strabismus** is a deviation of the eye in which the angle of deviation does *not* vary with the direction of gaze or the fixating eye.

In **paralytic strabismus** the deviation of the eye becomes greater as the eye is moved in the direction of function of the paretic muscle.

There are a number of possible causes of a concomitant strabismus. These include defects of innervation, refraction, and accommodation plus a genetic predisposition as well as a large group in which the cause is unknown. Common causes are imbalance of the near reflex (accommodative strabismus) and unilateral reduced vision in an infant or child.

By about age 7 years the accommodative and fusion reflexes are set. Muscle imbalance before this age results in concomitant strabismus. Muscle imbalance after this age is usually paralytic in type. It is not always easy to classify strabismus as concomitant or paralytic.

Concomitant strabismus does not usually produce the complaint of double vision. When a patient has a latent strabismus (phoria) and, because of fatigue or a debilitating illness, presents with a manifest strabismus (tropia), he may complain of the sudden onset of double vision. If the distance between the two images is the same in every direction of gaze, this is not paralytic.

In concomitant strabismus *monocular* eye movements are full in all directions, the angle of deviation is the same in all directions of gaze, and the primary and secondary deviations are identical irrespective of which eye fixates.

Paralytic Strabismus

In a paralytic strabismus the *secondary* squint position or secondary deviation of the *normal* eye is greater than the *primary* squint position of the paretic eye.

Example: With a left lateral rectus palsy, the left eye deviates from the midline while the right eye fixes straight ahead. The left eye might be adducted 5 degrees. If the right eye is then shielded, the left eye fixes in the straight-ahead position and the right eye adducts 10 degrees. This is the **secondary deviation**.

The more recent the paralytic squint, the greater is the angle of deviation in the various gaze positions. A single extraocular muscle palsy is easiest to recognize on the day it occurs. As time goes by, some degree of concomitance occurs. This will involve (a) overreaction of the yoke muscle (ie, the right lateral rectus and the left medial rectus are yoke muscles; each extraocular muscle has a yoke, or partner, muscle of the other eye); (b) contracture of the unopposed ipsilateral agonist of the paretic muscle; and (c) underfunction of the contralateral yoke muscle related to the agonist in (b).

MISCELLANEOUS

Abnormal Head Posture

In the analysis of any patient with double vision, the way he holds his head may be helpful. When a head turn is present, the patient turns his head into the field of action of the paretic muscle; that is, if the left lateral rectus muscle is paretic, he turns his chin to his left shoulder. As he faces you, he adducts the left eye and abducts the right eye. He then sees only one doctor—and that is enough for anyone, especially if he is sick! However, the patient may do the opposite—in our example, he would turn his chin to his right shoulder and look at you from the nasal corner of his right eye, with the left eye as abducted as the weak lateral rectus will take it.

The separation of the two images is so great and the false one is on such a peripheral aspect of the retina that it is suppressed.

Eye Patch

The patient almost always covers or closes the paretic eye. She may be a myasthenic with *multiple* weak extraocular muscles for whom the side of the patch is of no lateralizing help. However, if a single muscle or two muscles of the same eye are at fault, the closed eye is usually the paretic eye.

Ask the patient to take off the patch, to keep both eyes open, and to put her head in the position where there is *no* double vision. If her chin comes up and her head goes back into extension, she has weak eye elevators. Side-to-side movement has already been discussed. The head is *tilted* with the ear to the shoulder most commonly with *oblique* muscle palsies. With a superior oblique palsy the head is turned and tilted away from the weak side.

Monocular Diplopia

Monocular diplopia can result from opacities in the vitreous, lens, or cornea or from a dislocated lens (Marfan's syndrome) as well as astigmatism and early cataract. There are well-documented cases of occipital cortex injury resulting in monocular diplopia and quadruple vision with both eyes open.

CAUSES AND SITES OF LESIONS OF THE SIXTH CRANIAL NERVE

1. *Within the pons*, causes include
   a. Multiple sclerosis
   b. Infarct

    c. Mass (eg, glioma or tuberculoma)
    d. Wernicke's syndrome

Look for *ipsilateral*

- Seventh nerve lesion
- Gaze palsy
- Horner's syndrome
- Facial hypesthesia
- Internuclear ophthalmoplegia
- Ataxia

Look for *contralateral*

- Hemiparesis
- Nystagmus (possibly in more than one direction)
- Hemisensory pain and temperature loss in the trunk or limbs

  2. *At the base of the brain*, causes include
    a. Acoustic neuroma
    b. Meningitis
    c. Subarachnoid hemorrhage
    d. Compression of an aneurysm or anomalous vessel
    e. Basal meningioma
    f. Nasopharyngeal carcinoma
    g. Chordoma
    h. Wegener's granulomatosis

Look for signs of involvement of the fifth, seventh, and eighth cranial nerves.

  3. *In relation to the petrous portion of the temporal bone*, causes include
    a. Infection, fracture, or tumor of the petrous bone

Look for pain, paresthesia, or hyperesthesia of the face (same side) and deafness.

  4. *In the cavernous sinus/superior orbital fissure*, causes include
    a. Aneurysm (carotid)
    b. Carotid—cavernous fistula (trauma)
    c. Tumor—pituitary, meningioma, or nasopharyngeal carcinoma

    d. Tolosa-Hunt syndrome
    e. Cavernous sinus thrombosis
    f. Mucormycosis (in diabetics)
    g. Herpes zoster

Look for signs of involvement of the third and fourth cranial nerves as well as first and second divisions of the fifth.

5. *In the orbit*, causes include
    a. Tumor
    b. Trauma
6. *Common and not so common causes, but with an uncertain site*, include
    a. Postviral infection (especially in children)
    b. Diabetes
    c. Hypertension
    d. Postlumbar puncture or myelogram
    e. Increased intracranial pressure
    f. Migraine
    g. Arteritis or angiitis of sarcoidosis
    h. Fisher variant of Guillain-Barré syndrome
7. *Other causes of abduction defect* include
    a. Thyroid ophthalmopathy
    b. Myasthenia gravis
    c. Orbital pseudotumor
    d. Trauma
    e. Duane's syndrome
    f. Convergence spasm

CAUSES AND SITES OF LESIONS OF THE OCULOMOTOR NERVE

Remember that the *right* superior rectus is supplied by part of the nucleus of the *left* oculomotor nerve and vice versa. There is only *one* midline nuclear structure that supplies *both* the right and left levator palpebrae superioris muscles.

1. *Within the midbrain*, causes include
    a. *Complete unilateral* nuclear lesion, although it probably does not exist
    b. Partial unilateral (nuclear or fascicular) infarction or hemorrhage, demyelination, or tumor

Look for contralateral

- Hemiparkinsonian signs
- Hemihypesthesia
- Hemiparesis in the face, arm, and leg
- Ataxia and possibly tremor

2. *Interpeduncular* causes include
   a. Aneurysm (in the posterior communicating artery or basilar artery)
   b. Meningitis
   c. Infarction (in diabetics the *pupil* is usually *normal* and the infarction is often painful)
3. *At the edge of the tentorium* (herniation of the uncus from an expanding intracranial mass), causes include
   a. Contralateral upper motor neuron signs
   b. Deteriorating vital signs
   c. Progressing drowsiness
4. *Within the cavernous sinus*, causes are the same as those for the abducens nerve (see above).
5. *Within the orbit*, causes are the same as those for the abducens nerve. Additionally, thyroid ophthalmopathy with tethered medial rectus may be a cause, that is, defective *abduction* is seen, and with inferior rectus restriction defective elevation is seen.
6. *Common and not so common causes, but with an uncertain site*, include
   a. Migraine
   b. Diabetes (common)
   c. Hypertension
   d. Arteritis
   e. Collagen-vascular disease

CAUSES AND SITES OF LESIONS OF THE TROCHLEAR NERVE

The causes and sites of lesions of the trochlear nerve are the same as those of the oculomotor nerve. The most common cause is trauma and the next is diabetes. The latter probably produces an ischemic infarction of the nerve trunk.

Ptosis and the Pupils: *Myasthenia Gravis and Other Diseases of the Eye and Eyelid Muscles*

5

PTOSIS

Ptosis is often the greatest abnormality in familial, chronic progressive external ophthalmoplegia (CPEO).

In other diseases ptosis is often the presenting (and only) symptom. If it is bilateral, long-standing, and familial, the diagnosis is probably CPEO (see below).

If it is unilateral, recent, partial, and the only abnormality, the problem is more difficult to diagnose.

The space between the lids (palpebral fissure) varies. Increased sympathetic function increases the space and so does adduction of the eye in many people. With the eyes in the primary position, the space is about 7–12 mm in the vertical midline. The cornea is about 10.5 mm in vertical diameter; the upper lid usually covers the top 0.5–1 mm, and the bottom lid touches the lower limbus.

Buy an inexpensive transparent plastic ruler marked in millimeters and start to measure the fissure every time you have the chance.

Blepharospasm or Ptosis?

Blepharospasm is eye closure resulting from a **contraction** of the orbicularis oculi muscle. Ptosis is partial or complete eye closure caused by **paresis** or **paralysis** of the levator palpebrae muscle or the superior tarsal muscle.

Blepharospasm may be a result of some painful or irritating ocular disease, or it may be voluntary to abolish the false image of diplopia. It may also be a dystonia, that is, an involuntary movement because of organic disease, in this case always bilateral. When unilateral, how is blepharospasm distinguished from ptosis? In **blepharospasm** the eyebrow is pulled down *below* the superior orbital margin. In **ptosis** it is on the margin or *above*. If above, the forehead is wrinkled as the patient uses his frontalis to compensate for the drooping lid.

Is Ptosis Part of a Third Nerve Palsy or of a Horner's Syndrome?

If there is a big pupil on the side of the ptosis, with or without the appropriate extraocular muscle palsies, the diagnosis is a third nerve lesion. If there is a small pupil on the same side, it is a Horner's syndrome (see below under "Pupils," with regard to the response of the pupil to decreased illumination in Horner's syndrome). A third nerve lesion can cause complete ptosis; a Horner's syndrome cannot. On upward gaze, the ptosis of a third nerve palsy does not change; however, if it is part of a Horner's syndrome, it will diminish.

If the pupils are equal, look at the lower lid. The inferior tarsal muscle (which pulls the lower lid down) is paretic in a Horner's syndrome and *the lower lid is higher than the normal lower lid*. It covers more of the limbus at 6 o'clock.

Bilateral ptosis without the other signs of either third nerve or sympathetic lesions has been seen following basilar artery infarction and ischemia. The ptosis was an isolated ocular finding. The pupils and eye movements were normal, and the patients were alert.

PUPILS

Pupillary size, equality between right and left, and pupil responses to various stimuli in the *conscious* and *comatose* patient are prime physical signs.

Size

Pupil size depends on the light, the near reaction, and sympathetic and parasympathetic tone. Newborns and the elderly have smaller pupils than do youths. Schizophrenic patients and frightened people have big pupils. Blue-eyed people have bigger pupils than brown-eyed people, and myopic people also have larger pupils. Use a transparent plastic ruler to measure pupil size.

The pupils in young people often constrict and dilate in a repetitive rhythmic way. This is hippus and is normal. Its absence, however, is also normal. Most pupils in the examining room are 2–5 mm in diameter.

Equality

Most people have pupils of equal size. About 15–20% of patients have unequal pupils (anisocoria) that cannot be explained, but the difference is usually not more than 1 mm. If the difference remains constant in both bright and dim illumination, it is not significant. If the *difference* in size changes with the illumination, then disease is present. The small pupil of a Horner's syndrome will not *dilate* in dim light as much as the pupil of the other normal eye. The larger pupil of a partial third nerve palsy will not *constrict* as much as the normal pupil when the patient is in a bright light. Therefore, measure pupil sizes in average room light, dimness, and bright light. (Practice this first with classmates or patients with equal pupils.)

Two things that do *not* cause unequal pupils are

1. Unilateral or bilateral diminished or absent visual acuity or peripheral visual field defects
2. Differences in refractive errors between the two eyes

Pupils are displaced slightly to the nasal side of the center of the irises and are round. Eccentric pupils are not necessarily abnormal, and irregularities of shape are usually caused by trauma.

How to Examine the Pupils

Light Reaction   Examine the patient while she is sitting, with moderate background illumination. Inspect and compare the pupils while your flashlight is held vertically, pointing up, below the eye, and just in front of the patient's cheek.

Then ask the patient to look at the far wall and direct a bright light at first one and then the other eye. Be careful not to illuminate the two eyes at the same time.

Both pupils should react to the light in *either* eye with equal speed and to the same degree. This tests the second cranial nerve and other parts of the visual pathways (afferent) and the pupillary fibers of the third cranial nerve (efferent).

Direct and Consensual Light Reaction   A *direct* pupil response to light means that the right pupil constricts when the right eye is exposed to a bright light. A *consensual* response means that the right pupil constricts when the left eye is exposed to a bright light, and vice versa.

If the right eye has a normal direct response and an abnormal consensual response, the lesion is in the afferent pathway of the left eye. If the right eye has an abnormal direct response and a normal consensual response, the lesion is in the afferent pathway of the right eye. If the right eye has neither a direct nor a consensual response, the lesion is in the efferent pathway on the right (third nerve palsy). A lesion at the apex of the right orbit involving both efferent and afferent limbs of the reflex may also abolish direct and consensual responses for the right eye.

Near Reaction If the light reflex works, so will the near reflex. If one or both pupils do *not* react to light, ask the patient to look at the far wall and then at the tip of your pencil, which should be 5–10 cm in front of his nose. If his visual acuity is seriously compromised, ask the patient to look at the tip of his own finger held in front of his nose.

Look for two things: bilateral constriction of the pupils as the patient changes his gaze from far to near and convergence of the eyes. Accommodation also occurs. This increases curvature of the lens and is a result of contraction of the ciliary muscle and loosening of the suspensory ligament.

If the right eye has a *sluggish* direct pupillary response to light, relative to the direct left response, but has a brisk near response, the lesion is in the right afferent limb of the light reflex.

Afferent Pupil Defect, Swinging Flashlight Test, and Marcus Gunn Pupil Take, for example, the case of a patient with retrobulbar neuritis of the right optic nerve. His vision is 20/80 right, 20/20 left; peripheral fields are full; and the retina, optic nerve head, and media are all normal. Examine his pupil responses in dim illumination. Shine a strong light into his *left eye only*. Both pupils constrict as expected. Shield the left eye from light and shine the light into the *right eye only*. The right pupil seems to constrict momentarily and then dilates widely, as does the left. Swing the light back to the left eye only and again both constrict.

The high-intensity light-induced impulses from the left eye have their normal influence on the two pretectal and Edinger-Westphal nuclei. The efferent systems (third nerves) are normal, so both pupils constrict. However, when the light is directed into the right eye, the pupil changes from the constriction of a *normal consensual* light reaction to the relative dilatation of a low-intensity *direct* reaction. This low-intensity response is caused by diminished conduction through the diseased afferent system of the right eye. The left pupil also dilates as the consensual response in this eye is determined by the afferent system on the right.

Causes and Types of Abnormal Pupils

Argyll-Robertson Pupils Argyll-Robertson pupils are usually bilateral and result from tertiary syphilis of the nervous system, diabetes, or the late signs of bilateral tonic pupils (see the section on "Adie's Syndrome"). The pupils are *small*, irregular, and unequal. They do not react to light, they do react to near vision, they respond poorly to mydriatics, and they do not dilate in the dark. However, they can be made to constrict even more by the use of miotics. The poor light response and good near response may be relative; that is, the light response need not be absent, but is much less evident than the near response. Visual acuity is not impaired.

Horner's Syndrome Horner's syndrome, or oculosympathetic palsy (unilateral), presents with abnormalities of the *eyelids* as described in the section on "Ptosis." The pupil is small and round with good response to light and near. The difference between normal and abnormal pupil size in the *dark* is even greater; that is, the pupil on the side of the lesion dilates later and less. A lesion of the sympathetic fibers can be in the brain stem, cervical cord, apex of the lung, carotid sheath, or orbit.

Additional signs are apparent enophthalmos and a warm, dry, nonsweating, ipsilateral face. A number of pharmacological agents can be used to aid the diagnosis and localize the lesion as central, preganglionic, or postganglionic.

Horner's syndrome, with pain in the eye and ipsilateral face and forehead, has been reported in dissection of the carotid artery and with cluster headaches with a normal carotid artery.

Oculomotor Nerve Lesion (Unilateral) Other features of the unilateral oculomotor nerve lesion are as described above. The pupil is mid-dilated. There is *no* response to light or near, and the difference in pupil size is greater in the *light* (in contrast with Horner's syndrome). Mydriatics and miotics are both effective. Diabetic oculomotor nerve palsies usually have normal pupils, and lesions can be painful.

Adie's Syndrome Adie's syndrome, or tonic pupil (which may be unilateral or asymmetrically bilateral), is also known as "the big, slow pupil." The condition presents as an enlarged pupil that either does not react to light or eventually constricts after being exposed to very bright light for 15–20 min. It eventually constricts for near after a similarly long effort. Redilatation is just as protracted. The difference in the pupil sizes is best seen in the *light*.

The pupils respond to mydriatics and miotics and demonstrate **denervation supersensitivity**. This means that the tonic pupil will constrict from 2.5% solution of Mecholyl or 0.125% pilocarpine. Normal pupils do not respond to these weak solutions.

Accommodation is just as slow as the light response and may be the presenting complaint. When the deep tendon reflexes are diminished or absent, the syndrome is called Holmes-Adie. The cause is unknown.

Benign Anisocoria Usually a young adult with benign anisocoria reports a difference in pupil size. The longer it has been present, the less likely it is to be important. Ask for some old photographs of the patient, and examine them for pupil inequalities. The response to light and near in both eyes is normal, the *difference* in pupil size is no greater in dimness or light, mydriatics and miotics have a normal response, and there is no diagnosis.

The Factitious Big Pupil Sometimes proprietary eyedrops have impurities in them with atropine-like properties. Patients using ointments with atropine-like properties may inadvertently introduce them into the eye.

There is occasionally a deliberate atropine abuser. He or she is usually working or studying in a hospital and has some access to medications and is under pressure or stress of some kind. The patient presents with the biggest pupil you have ever seen. There is not a flicker of response to light or near. The difference is greatest in bright light, and neither mydriatics nor miotics change the pupil.

Keep the patient talking (about anything), get the whole story, change the environment (if a medical student or nurse, keep him off the wards for the next 3 days if possible), and reexamine the eye daily for 3 consecutive days. If this big pupil is caused by medication, each day its response to light and near will be a little better and your chances of getting the full history improve. Pilocarpine will not constrict an atropinized pupil; it will, however, constrict an Adie's pupil.

Midbrain Lesions With midbrain lesions the pupils are large, particularly if the lesion involves the parasympathetic fibers of the third nerve. If the midbrain is totally interrupted, including the sympathetic fibers, the pupils are big, but less so.

Carotid Artery Occlusion (Unilateral) An enlarged pupil ipsilateral to the occlusion has been reported in atheroma and Takayasu's disease. The pupil reacts poorly to light (direct and indirect) and near. The explanation is probably ischemic atrophy of the iris, rather than nerve disease.

Pontine Miosis (Bilateral) The classic sign of pontine infarction or hemorrhage is small (1- to 1.5-mm) pupils. They will constrict to light if a bright enough stimulus is used and if examined through a magnifying glass.

ACCOMMODATION AND CONVERGENCE

For near vision the eyes converge (ie, turn toward the midline), the pupils constrict, and the lenses thicken. In order to complete an examination, the patient must cooperate. When the simultaneous contractions of the two medial recti produce convergence, they have a different central connection than when either is being used for conjugate lateral gaze in conjunction with its appropriate yoke muscle, that is, the contralateral lateral rectus.

Failing accommodation is most commonly related to aging, as the lens becomes less resilient. The parasympathetic nerve fibers subserving accommodation, as well as those subserving the pupillary near response, will be interrupted in a complete peripheral third nerve palsy.

The diabetic, out of control or of recent onset, can have a sudden increase in the refractive power of the lens; that is, a sudden improvement in near vision is as much a symptom as the reverse. Anticholinergic drugs commonly produce a complaint of blurred vision from diminished accommodation if taken in large enough doses.

Near Response

1. If the pupils react to light, they will react to near.
2. If the pupils do not react to light, it is important to know whether the near response is also abnormal.
3. If there is a defect in adduction, it is important to know whether or not convergence is present. (See the section on "Internuclear Ophthalmoplegia" in Chapter 7.) You can verify the patient's efforts to converge by the attendant miosis, which means she is trying.
4. In any bilateral paresis of external ocular muscles, convergence assessment is part of the examination that may help you localize and diagnose the lesion.
5. The sudden onset of diplopia, with eyes divergent, but with full monocular eye movements, is a **paresis of convergence**.
6. The periaqueduct syndrome, discussed in the section on "Parinaud's Syndrome" in Chapter 7, includes paresis of convergence.
7. Convergence excess looks like a unilateral or bilateral lateral rectus palsy. The patient is staring at the tip of his nose. This is often a hysterical disease. When you ask the patient to look laterally, which he says he cannot do, his pupils constrict, proving that he is overconverging. However, it can be organic following head injury and can be part of the periaqueduct syndrome.
8. Miscellaneous: The toxin of *Clostridium botulinum* can produce large, nonreacting pupils, paralysis of accommodation, ptosis, and extraocular muscle palsies. The patient is wide awake, with progressing respiratory distress. He may have vomited but is usually constipated. Diphtheria can produce paralysis of accommodation and also affects bulbar originating nerves and cardiac rhythm.

OTHER DISEASES WITH WEAKNESS OF THE EYE AND EYELID MUSCLES

Myasthenia Gravis

Myasthenia gravis is a common cause of ocular complaints, often diagnosed late. It may present as weakness of one muscle or one eye or any combination of muscles. The essence of the disease is excessive fatigability, that is, the patient cannot *sustain* upward gaze or *sustain* the upper lids in a fixed open position. Of all the possible combinations of myasthenic muscle weakness (eg, ocular, pharyngeal, or limb), **bilateral fluctuating undulating ptosis** is probably the most common.

Look at the patient's eyes and keep looking. She may blink three times with blinks of the same duration and the same interval between blinks, but she does not open as wide after each blink. Then, in the fourth blink, she keeps her eyes closed for 10–20 s. She is not sleeping and you are not that boring—when she finally opens her eyes after the long blink, her ptosis is less pronounced and you can see more of her eyes. She then has three or four of her usual blinks with her ptosis increasing and then has another long blink. You are looking at a patient with myasthenia gravis.

When the **eye opening muscles** are weak and the **eye closing muscles** are also weak, the diagnosis is almost always either myasthenia gravis or one of the CPEOs (see the following section). Therefore, when the patient has ptosis (you know the eye openers are weak) test the **eye closers**. The diagnosis of myasthenia gravis starts when you first consider it. There are immunological, neurophysiological, pharmacological, and therapeutic ways to help make the diagnosis, but it usually all starts when a *young woman* or an *old man* says, "My eyelids are drooping" or "I see double when I'm watching the late news on TV."

Chronic Progressive External Ophthalmoplegia

CPEO is actually a number of diseases. They have in common a *progressive*, *restricted* range of eye movements and *ptosis*. Some, however, have ptosis only. The patient may know nothing about this. Most of his family members look the same, the diseases are very chronic, and they usually do not cause diplopia. Often, an associated symptom unrelated to the abnormal ocular mobility brings the patient to the doctor. Included in this group of diseases are:

1. Oculopharyngeal dystrophy—Common in French Canadians, is autosomal dominant; ptosis is more marked than gaze limitations, and trouble swallowing is often the presenting complaint.
2. Myotonic dystrophy—Presents with action and percussion myotonia; weak neck (sternomastoid), temporal and masseter, and limb muscles; marked ptosis; and cataracts
3. Thyroid ocular myopathy—Patients commonly complain of diplopia, thyroid status may be normal, proptosis may be absent, and lid lag on downward gaze and inability to *elevate* the globe are the most common

signs. This myopathy commonly involves the **medial rectus muscle**, producing a secondary limited abduction that mimics a lateral rectus palsy.

The syndromes are

- Stephens—A positive family history of CPEO plus peripheral neuropathy and cerebellar ataxia
- Kearns-Sayre—Childhood onset of CPEO, retinal pigment degeneration, heart block plus progressive encephalopathy and sometimes cerebellar signs, short stature, and a negative family history
- Bassen-Kornzweig—Abetalipoproteinemia
- Chronic multiple sclerosis
- Chronic myasthenia gravis
- Myotubular myopathy

Nystagmus 6

Nystagmus is a rhythmic oscillation of the eye or eyes.

Nystagmus is usually a sign of disease in the posterior fossa or peripheral vestibular apparatus. However, the most rostral structure, when diseased enough that it can cause nystagmus, is the thalamus; the most caudal is the neural axis at the level of the craniocervical junction. The nature of the nystagmus may reveal the site of the lesion causing it; that is, nystagmus of the abducting eye *only* is always a result of intrinsic brain stem disease and vertical nystagmus is never vestibular in origin. In many cases other physical signs are used to determine the site of the nystagmus-producing lesion. In some patients the precise site of the lesion is unknown.

Alcohol and other drugs are a common cause of nystagmus and are the most common cause of transient coexisting horizontal and vertical nystagmus.

Nystagmus is classified into several types with considerable overlap: these include acquired or congenital; jerk or pendular; present with the eyes in the primary position or gaze-evoked; present or modified when the patient is upright, supine, prone, or with his head tilted; and present in the light or the dark.

TYPES OF NYSTAGMUS

Jerk

Jerk nystagmus is the most common type. When the patient is asked to follow the examiner's finger to the right, his eyes are seen to drift off the point of fixation (the finger) and back to the midline. They then snap back to the finger. The nystagmus is named from the direction of the *fast* (ie, correcting) movement, that is, right beating jerk nystagmus on right lateral gaze. In jerk nystagmus the two movements are never of the same *velocity*.

Pendular

In pendular nystagmus the movement of the eyes in one direction is at the same speed as the movement in the other direction. For this reason pendular nystagmus is not named right, left, and so on, but is named from the plane of the movement, that is, horizontal, vertical, or rotary. Pendular nystagmus can be **acquired** or *congenital*.

Gaze-Evoked

With the eyes in the primary position, no nystagmus is seen.

- Ask the patient to follow your finger in all the principal directions of gaze with the finger 60 cm from him and both eyes open.
- Have him do it again with one and then the other eye closed.
- Repeat the above with the finger close enough to the patient to make him converge while he looks in all the principal directions.

Nystagmus elicited from any of these procedures will be described as, for example, "bilateral left beating nystagmus on left lateral gaze," or whatever eye position is necessary to evoke it.

Primary Eye Position

When the patient looks straight ahead, nystagmus may be present. It can be **jerk** or **pendular**. When the former, it is often so fine that you need to watch a retinal vessel with your ophthalmoscope in order to see it. It may be vertical (fast component) or lateral. It may become coarser or vanish when the patient looks to either side.

Congenital

Pendular Congenital nystagmus is most commonly **pendular**. The history is of vital importance. The patient may "do something" (ie, consult a doctor) about his jumping eyes for the first time at age 16. Diminished visual acuity is a common but *not* causal accompanying feature. Nystagmus is usually horizontal, is always in both eyes, and diminishes with convergence. It will change from pendular in the primary position to jerk on lateral gaze. These patients often have a head tremor that only appears or worsens when they try to read. The patient will usually have a head and eye position where the nystagmus is least or absent, known as the **null position**.

There is often rhythm to congenital pendular nystagmus. The patient will have five or six oscillations of the eyes, followed by a pause of 1–2 s, during which the movements almost vanish, and then the oscillations resume. (See the section on "Optokinetic Nystagmus," below, and its effect on congenital nystagmus, also described below.)

Probably the most common cause of nystagmus is congenitally poor vision in both eyes from any cause.

Latent Latent nystagmus is also congenital. When the patient has both eyes open and the eyes in the primary position, there is no nystagmus. When either eye is covered, both eyes develop marked **jerk** nystagmus, fast phase to the side of the uncovered eye. Visual acuity is decreased when one eye is covered. Many patients with this type of nystagmus have a strabismus.

LESION SITES

In general, when the patient looks in the direction of the fast movement, the amplitude of the nystagmus becomes greater. The *fast* component of nystagmus is dependent on the integrity of the *opposite* cerebral hemisphere, basal ganglia, and diencephalon; that is, an acute destructive right vestibular lesion will produce conjugate ocular deviation to the right and nystagmus to the left. If the patient has an additional right middle cerebral artery territory infarct, there will be no nystagmus.

Brain Stem, Cerebellar Nuclei, and Their Connections

1. **Jerk** (the most common type of nystagmus resulting from acquired disease)
   a. May be in the abducting eye only, and the intensity increases when looking in the direction of the fast phase. It is often easily exhausted and can be three or four coarse beats in the abducting eye only and then stop.
   b. May be equal in the two eyes
   c. May be associated with limited adduction of the other eye as part of an internuclear ophthalmoplegia (see Chapter 7)
   d. Downbeat—May be difficult to see in the primary eye position as described in the section on primary eye position nystagmus, above. Will become coarser on conjugate downward gaze and much coarser (while remaining downbeating) on lateral conjugate gaze to either side. Usually vanishes on conjugate upward gaze. Usually increased when posture changes from upright to supine. Responsible lesions are usually cerebellar herniation or degeneration or Arnold-Chiari malformation.
   e. Upbeat (two types)—One type is present and easily seen in the primary position and will increase with upward gaze and decrease with downward gaze; the lesion is in the anterior vermis of the cerebellum. The other type of upbeat nystagmus is difficult to see in the primary position and is paradoxical in that it increases with downward gaze. The responsible lesion may be in the tegmental gray matter at the pontine-medullary or pontine-midbrain junction. Both upbeating and downbeating nystagmus may be modified by head tilting or may appear only on head tilting.

2. **Rotary** only
3. **Mixed rotary and jerk**
4. **Acquired pendular**—Present in many directions (ie, vertical or horizontal) and may be different in the two eyes. It is often accompanied by signs of disease of nearby structures, for example, slurred speech, ataxia of the limbs and gait, diplopia, and tremor.

Vestibular (Peripheral or End Organ) Lesions

Nystagmus resulting from vestibular lesions occurs in one direction only, always *away* from the lesion. It is usually mixed, lateral, and rotary. It is never **vertical** or **rotary** only, is reduced by visual fixation, and is always accompanied by marked vertigo and usually by tinnitus and hearing loss.

Diencephalon

This is a seesaw, pendular nystagmus with no fast component. There are conjugate rotational eye movements plus a bizarre vertical movement. The eye that rotates inward rises as the eye that rotates outward drops. The vertical seesaw movements may be elicited in downward gaze only. It can be congenital. The site of the lesion responsible for this type of nystagmus is not firmly established.

ASSOCIATED SIGNS AND SYMPTOMS

1. With nystagmus of brain stem or cerebellar origin,
   a. Ataxia, dysarthria, diplopia, internuclear ophthalmoplegia (see Chapter 7), other cranial nerve lesions, long tract motor and sensory signs
   b. Vertigo, absent or relatively mild and improved by lying still with the eyes closed
2. With nystagmus of vestibular origin,
   a. Vertigo and vomiting are intense, onset of both is abrupt, and the patient usually cannot be induced to move or get up; the patient feels that the *environment* is rotating *away* from the side of the lesion.
   b. Other signs of eighth cranial nerve dysfunction are present (see Chapter 9).
   c. There are no signs of brain stem or cerebellar disease but the eyes are forced to the side of the lesion.
   d. There is usually a history of tinnitus or reduced hearing.
   e. If the patient can be induced to stand and walk, he staggers *to* the side of the lesion.

MISCELLANEOUS

End-Point Nystagmus

Normal, seen at the extremes of lateral gaze, end-point nystagmus is of the small, irregular jerk type, best seen in the abducting eye. It is more marked and common in association with even minor alcohol intake.

Convergence Nystagmus

Convergence will usually dampen congenital nystagmus and peripheral vestibular nystagmus. Nystagmus seen only during convergence can be part of the dorsal midbrain syndrome.

Rebound Nystagmus

With this condition, the patient looks, for example, to the left and has left beating jerk nystagmus. It stops and when he moves his eyes back to the primary position, nystagmus reappears as right beating nystagmus in the primary position. After a few seconds it stops again. This signifies intrinsic brain stem/cerebellar disease. It is important to watch the patient's eyes as they come back to the primary position, as this may be the *only* position in which you see any nystagmus.

Periodic Alternating Nystagmus

This is an uncommon, startling type of nystagmus. The patient will have a spontaneous constant jerk nystagmus in one direction; it will stop after some seconds and, after a short interval of no nystagmus, will resume in the opposite direction. This alternating goes on constantly. It is significant in a number of acquired and congenital posterior fossa disorders. It can occur in otherwise normal people.

Convergence-Retraction Nystagmus

On attempting to look upward, rapid repetitive convergent movements with retraction of the eyes occur. The lesion is in the midbrain (see the section on "Parinaud's Syndrome" in Chapter 7).

Voluntary Nystagmus

Voluntary nystagmus is not a true nystagmus. It is a very rapid, usually side-to-side, oscillation or rotation with the eyes in the primary position and with voluntary overconvergence. Like the ability to voluntarily move one's ears, a few of us can do it, but most of us cannot. The person with voluntary nystagmus can keep it up for only a few seconds at a time. This is not a manifestation of disease. When present in a medical student, it can win small wagers from other medical students, as in "Did you know I can have nystagmus any time I want to?"

Optokinetic Nystagmus

Optokinetic nystagmus (OKN) is also referred to as "railroad" nystagmus. If you have ridden on a train and watched the utility poles go by, you have had OKN in the direction (ie, fast phase) that the train is moving.

- Clinically, patients are tested for this by having them watch a revolving drum that has alternating black and white vertical stripes.
- At the bedside you may use a cloth 1.0-m measuring tape; however, if you want even better contrast, buy a roll of black electrician's tape and stick 15-mm pieces onto your 1.0-m cloth tape, 15 mm apart. Draw it through your fingers from left to right, asking the patient to look at a number on the tape as it appears and follow it until it disappears and then look at another number and follow it.

Repeat the process from right to left. Watch the patient's eyes. For a few seconds after the tape has stopped moving or the drum has stopped rotating, spontaneous nystagmus is seen.

Most people have OKN. The **slow** phase is in the *following* direction, and the **rapid** phase is the direction the tape is coming *from*. It can be evoked in the horizontal or vertical plane.

Who Does Not Have OKN?

1. The *drowsy* or *uncooperative* patient, who looks "through" the tape. He has no OKN to the right, left, up, or down.
2. The patient with a *defect of fixation*. Fixation requires
   a. A functioning macula and normal visual acuity
   b. Contours or contrast in the object being seen; that is, you cannot fix your vision on a perfectly cloudless blue sky
   c. The object seen must arouse the attention of the subject
3. The patient with a gaze palsy (see Chapter 7). OKN is absent in the direction of the gaze palsy.
4. The patient with a *homonymous field defect*—absolute or inattention— may have absent OKN to the side of the defect. This is most consistent when the lesion is in the *middle* or *posterior* part of the **optic radiation**, that is, the parietal lobe. If OKN is equal to the right and left and a homonymous defect is present, the lesion is probably in the occipital lobe.

5. The patient with congenital nystagmus (see the section earlier in this chapter). The OKN response in most of these patients is the opposite of what one would expect and is known as "inverted." The OKN response can be used to differentiate acquired from congenital nystagmus; that is, if the patient has vestibular nystagmus to her right and a tape is presented moving to her left, the OKN will be added to the vestibular nystagmus. If her nystagmus stops or reverses its direction after she looks at the tape, her nystagmus is congenital. This is a reliable way to differentiate congenital from acquired nystagmus and may save a patient from expensive, possibly dangerous, and needless, investigations.

Conjugate Gaze Palsies and Forced Conjugate Deviation

7

Conjugate gaze palsies or forced conjugate gaze may result from disease of the cerebrum, diencephalon, brain stem, cerebellum, or peripheral labyrinth apparatus.

Conjugate gaze palsies do not cause double vision. Patients usually do not know there is anything amiss with the way their eyes move in tandem. A decreased level of consciousness frequently accompanies a gaze palsy or forced conjugate gaze of acute onset.

When a patient has a conjugate gaze palsy to the left, he cannot look to the left of the midline with either eye but he does not have paresis of the left lateral rectus muscle or of the right medial rectus.

There is more than one way to demonstrate a gaze palsy, and the method is important; that is, if the patient cannot look to the left *when asked*, can he *pursue* an object moving to his left, or can he *fix* on a stationary object in front of him and keep looking at it as his chin is rotated to his right shoulder? Will his eyes move conjugately with *stimulation* of the labyrinth with hot or cold water? (See the section on eighth cranial nerve examination in Chapter 9.) Do his eyes respond normally to doll's eye testing (see below)? Therefore, a gaze palsy may be **voluntary**, **pursuit**, or **reflex** with different anatomical implications (supratentorial, brain stem, or peripheral).

Forced conjugate deviations are usually caused by acute lesions in seriously ill and often stuporous patients. All the centers concerned with conjugate gaze have opposing centers that have the opposite function. If the right cerebral hemisphere center concerned with conjugate gaze to the left is suddenly destroyed by a hemorrhage, the eyes will be forced to the right temporarily by the now unopposed left hemisphere center. Forced conjugate gaze is the result of either destruction or irritation of a nervous system gaze center or of a labyrinth lesion.

SUPRATENTORIAL GAZE "CENTERS"

Anterior, or Frontal, or Volitional, Saccadic Center

The caudal part of the middle frontal gyrus (part of Brodmann's area 8) is concerned with voluntary eye movements and is independent of visual stimuli. If the lesion is

1. *Irritative*, that is, epileptic seizure, the eyes and head will turn to the opposite side. This phenomenon has been reproduced experimentally, although the direction of the turn is not to the *opposite* side 100% of the time.
2. *Destruction* of the frontal cortex or its connections through the internal capsule, the eyes are *forced*, by the opposite healthy cortex, to the side of the lesion and away from the side of the paretic arm and leg. As the lesion becomes chronic, the eyes will again be in the primary position and will move to the side of the lesion, but for a time will not cross the midline to the side of the paretic arm and leg. In short, the *stroke* patient will *not* look toward his paretic arm and leg, whereas the *convulsing* patient *must* look toward his twitching arm and leg (usually).

To determine that the lesion is in the *hemisphere* and not the brain stem,

- Rapidly turn the patient's head to the side of the normal arm and leg and you will see her eyes move conjugately to the side of the paresis (this is the doll's eye test; see the section on "The Doll's Eye Test and Caloric Testing").
- Irrigate the external auditory canal on the side of the abnormal arm and leg with cold water and the eyes will deviate to that side (see the section on examination of the eighth cranial nerve in Chapter 9).
- If the patient is alert enough to cooperate, have her fix her gaze at your finger (or her own) about 0.5 m in front of her. Ask her to keep staring at the finger as you rotate her head away from her paretic arm and leg. If the eyes stay fixed on the stationary finger, they will conjugately move to the side of the hemiparesis.

If the cause of the gaze palsy is in the *brain stem*, these three procedures will not produce conjugate gaze movement.

It is often difficult to tell whether a patient has a conjugate gaze palsy to one side of the midline, or a hemianopic field defect on the same side (he may have both; see the following section on the occipital eye center).The difficulty may be compounded because the patient is obtunded or dysphasic or both.

The presence of a field defect can be inferred by the following method:

- Bring your hand rapidly up to the patient's eyes from the side of his head in a threatening gesture.
- If he consistently blinks when the hand comes from one side but not from the other, he is probably hemianopic on the latter.
- If he blinks on both sides, he has a gaze palsy only and full visual fields.

Patients with conjugate gaze palsy from vascular disease of the anterior gaze "center" or its connections usually recover full eye movements. The recovery of the gaze palsy is usually much better than recovery of the paretic arm and leg.

Posterior, or Occipital, or Following, Smooth Pursuit Center

This center (approximately Brodmann's area 18) is less well defined than the anterior center, and lesions here are less common.

Destruction of the occipital eye center causes deviation of the eyes toward the lesion, and stimulation causes deviation away from the side of the lesion.

This center is concerned with following, largely involuntary, movements of the eyes. When diseased, the eyes will move in response to frontal, labyrinth, and doll's eye stimuli, but will not *follow* a moving object. The loss of conjugate gaze is almost always accompanied by a hemianopic field defect ipsilateral to the gaze palsy plus defective optokinetic nystagmus.

Summary

A lesion of the frontal gaze center prevents the patient from moving his eyes, on command, to the side opposite the lesion. He can *follow* an object to this side, however, provided that he will fix on it. A lesion of the occipital gaze center prevents the patient from following an object to the side opposite the lesion.

"WRONG WAY" CONJUGATE DEVIATION

Acute destructive lesions (hemorrhage) in the medial aspect of the thalamus on one side can result in a hemiparesis of the contralateral half of the body and the eyes conjugately forced *to* the side of the paresis.

CEREBELLAR GAZE PALSY

Cerebellar gaze palsy is seen with an acute unilateral cerebellar lesion. The eyes are deviated in the opposite direction. Ocular responses to labyrinth stimulation are normal.

DOWNWARD GAZE

Forced

With forced downward gaze the patient seems to be looking at his nose. He is usually comatose, there is some **convergence** as well as the fixed downward gaze, and his pupils are miotic. The most common cause is thalamic hemorrhage with extension into the midbrain. In acute Parinaud's syndrome, the eyes may be in a fixed downward position (see the section on "Paralysis," below). This physical sign has also been found, however, in patients with raised intracranial pressure and has been reversed when this was corrected. Doll's eye movement (in this case vertical, moving the patient's chin to his chest) results in no change in eye position.

Paralysis of Downward Gaze

Paralysis of downward gaze is an uncommon finding. It may exist as a congenital and familial finding. When an acquired sign, the lesion is likely to be destruction of the posterior thalamus or lesions of mesencephalic periaqueduct gray matter, ventral to the aqueduct. Loss of downward gaze may be part of Parinaud's syndrome and progressive supranuclear palsy. Difficulty with reading is often an early symptom.

UPWARD GAZE

Paralysis of Upward Gaze

Many people over 65 years of age and most patients with parkinsonism have defective, symptomless loss of conjugate upward gaze. This is evident on command and following. However, if they fix on a stationary object at eye level and the chin is depressed to the chest, the eyes will move upward.

Bilateral lesions of the pretectum will produce an upward gaze palsy.

BELL'S PHENOMENON

Bell's phenomenon is the normal turning up and out of the eye when a person closes his eyes. This is obvious in a patient with a seventh nerve palsy, as the eye on the paralyzed side cannot close and the movement of the globe is visible. It has some application in the assessment of patients with defective upward gaze.

> To elicit the phenomenon, have the patient sit facing you. Tell him to close his eyes as tightly as he can and resist your attempt to force them open. You can overcome his orbicularis oculi and you will see the globe turned up and out.

This is *normal*, and *almost* all people have it. The pathway for the reflex between the orbicularis oculi and the extraocular muscles is at brain stem level. Therefore, if a patient with defective upward gaze to command or on following has a normal Bell's phenomenon, the lesion is above the brain stem. Disease of the temporoparietal region can produce an abnormal Bell's phenomenon. The eyes will deviate laterally away from the side of the cerebral lesion.

PARINAUD'S SYNDROME

Parinaud's syndrome (also known as dorsal midbrain syndrome, or sylvian aqueduct syndrome) results from a lesion (glioma, hydrocephalus, germinoma, **pinealoma**, or vascular disease) of the supranuclear tectal or pretectal areas.

Signs consist of paresis of upward gaze and retraction nystagmus or convergence nystagmus on attempted upward gaze. There may be lid retraction or ptosis.

The pupils are enlarged and react poorly to light, but have normal near response. Convergence may be absent or in spasm. Downward gaze may also be defective, and vertical diplopia is common. Most patients will have papilledema. Upward optokinetic nystagmus is absent. The three most common components of the syndrome are

- Defective conjugate upward gaze
- Defective convergence
- Large pupils that respond more briskly to accommodation than to light

PONTINE RETICULAR FORMATION LESION

When unilateral, a permanent ipsilateral conjugate horizontal gaze palsy results. There is forced conjugate deviation to the opposite side only when the lesion is acute. When the lesion is rostral to the sixth nerve nucleus, labyrinth stimulation (cold) on the ipsilateral side will result in the eyes turning to that side. When the lesion is at the level of the sixth nerve nucleus, there is no response to labyrinth stimulation. Vertical movements and convergence are normal.

INTERNUCLEAR OPHTHALMOPLEGIA

Internuclear ophthalmoplegia (INO) results from a lesion in the medial longitudinal fasciculus (MLF) and may be demyelination, tumor, vascular disease, Wernicke's disease, systemic lupus, and others. Lesions at the anterior end of the MLF will have defective convergence. Posterior lesions have better medial rectus function on convergence than on gaze.

A unilateral INO will cause weakness of the medial rectus of the adducting ipsilateral eye varying from complete to partial as well as nystagmus of the abducting contralateral eye. The nystagmus of the abducting eye may be very coarse, slow, and easily exhausted. A bilateral INO reveals defective adduction to the right and left and nystagmus of the abducting eye on both directions of gaze. There may be nystagmus of the adducting eye as well. However, it is always of different and usually lesser amplitude and frequency than the abducting eye nystagmus.

THE "ONE-AND-A-HALF" SYNDROME

The "one-and-a-half" syndrome was first described by C. Miller Fisher ("Some Neuroophthalmological Observations." *J Neurol Neurosurg Psychiatry* 1967;**30**:383). It is a lesion (eg, vascular or demyelinating) of the pontine reticular formation and the ipsilateral medial longitudinal fasciculus.

Clinically, the ipsilateral eye has no movement in or out. The contralateral eye can abduct only but cannot cross the midline toward the nose.

(The pontine reticular formation lesion on the right, for example, will abolish conjugate gaze to the right for both eyes, the MLF lesion will abolish adduction for the right eye, and the only remaining lateral movement is abduction of the left eye.) Vertical movements are normal, as are the pupils.

SKEW DEVIATION

With skew deviation one eye is elevated and the other is depressed. The patient typically complains of diplopia. He may present with the elevated eye turned in. Skew deviation may be transient and may be the result of basilar artery ischemia, migraine, tumor, and trauma. Lesions may be in various parts of the brain stem and the cerebellum and the sign is not of precise localizing value.

THE DOLL'S EYE TEST AND CALORIC TESTING

In a comatose patient it is of great practical significance to be able to assess the integrity of the brain stem. The *doll's eye test* can help and is highly reliable. This test can be used in the conscious or unconscious patient.

The patient lies on his back without a pillow. Stand at the head of the bed. Hold the patient's eyes open with your thumbs or tape. Rapidly rotate the head to one side and hold it there. If the brain stem reflexes are intact, the eyes will move in the direction opposite the head rotation.

You can try this to the left and right, in flexion, and extension. If you are testing a conscious patient, ask him to fix on an object.

Caloric testing gives useful information when examining the unconscious patient.

Irrigate the external auditory canal with 20 mL of ice water (before doing this, see the section on "How to Test Vestibular Function" in Chapter 9). The eyes will turn toward that ear (or toward the opposite ear, if you use warm water).

If these simple tests show the appropriate eye movement, then the lesion causing the coma is not in the brain stem. When the brain stem is damaged, the eyes do not move.

Two cautions: If there is a possibility that **sedative drug overdose** or **freezing** may be contributing to the coma, both the doll's eye and caloric tests may lead you to think the brain stem reflexes are gone. They may not be. You cannot make a valid decision in these two conditions until you have examined reflex eye movements daily for several days.

PARALYSIS OF CONVERGENCE

In paralysis of convergence the patient complains of double vision with *greater separation* of the images when the object is *closer* to her than when it is farther away. This is the opposite of a lateral rectus palsy, in which the separation is greater when the object is farther away.

Further, the separation is the same *in all directions* of gaze, and testing of individual eye muscles, particularly the medial rectus, reveals a complete and full range of movement.

Inability to converge can be organic or functional. If you ask the patient to converge by looking at the tip of her own finger 30 cm from the tip of her nose, and there is no convergence but her pupils constrict, she has an organic convergence palsy. If the pupils do not constrict, you cannot say whether or not she has an organic lesion.

SUPRANUCLEAR CONVERGENCE PALSY

There is probably a cortical "center" concerned with convergence, and it is probably posterior somewhere in the occipital lobe. Head injuries to this region have been reported in association with convergence defects.

Cranial Nerves 1, 5, and 7　　8

FIRST CRANIAL NERVE (OLFACTORY NERVE)

Doctors get into trouble more from carelessness than from ignorance. The examinations of taste and smell are neglected more often than are any other parts of the nervous system.

How to Examine Smell

The test object is important. Do not use substances (eg, ammonia) that irritate the nasal mucosa. Granulated coffee, oil of peppermint, or oil of camphor will do.

> Ask the patient to close his eyes. Move the test substance toward him, under his nose, and then away from him. Ask him in advance to tell you when he smells something.

The objective is to see whether the patient will know when the test substance is under his nose. Can he tell the difference between this substance and nothing? The *name* of the substance is of no importance. Few people can identify ground coffee, peppermint, and camphor by smelling them, although almost every person can tell one from the other. Furthermore, the environment seems more important than the test substance; that is, almost everyone examined in a hospital says that peppermint is offensive and smells like some objectionable medicine. When smelled in a candy store, however, it is considered pleasant.

If **anosmia** exists, is the cause intranasal or intracranial? The common cold, allergic rhinitis, and hay fever can all abolish the sense of smell temporarily. Reexamine the patient if this may account for the anosmia.

Bilateral anosmia can be diagnosed easily and with certainty. However, because air diffuses throughout the nasal passages so quickly, a finding of **unilateral anosmia** is always suspect.

The most common cause of permanent anosmia is **head injury.** The lesion involves the 20 or so "nerve" fibers that leave the nasal mucosa and enter the skull through the cribriform plate of the ethmoid bone and join the olfactory bulb. These "nerves" can be sheared off with or without a fracture of the cribriform plate during a frontal or occipital injury. Because these fibers are unmyelinated central processes of olfactory sensory cells, they are not nerves and cannot repair themselves. The anosmia is permanent. The patient complains that she has lost her taste (most of what we call taste is really smell) and she is at risk because she cannot smell smoke, gas, or a skunk. One of the great pleasures in life (the ability to smell food, drink, and perfume) is gone forever to such patients.

Anterior fossa tumors, usually the meningioma, metastases to the skull, and nasopharyngeal carcinoma account for most of the other causes of anosmia. Look for frontal lobe signs, vision loss, and papilledema. The olfactory groove meningioma may be the explanation for the patient with chronic papilledema and no other obvious abnormalities. The diagnosis is obscure until the sense of smell is tested.

Dementia, old age, and central nervous system **sarcoidosis** can also cause anosmia.

When examining patients for the late effects of head injury, *always* test their sense of smell, irrespective of their complaints.

A chronic, distorted, unpleasant smell is a fairly common complaint and has no explanation. A short, strong, repeated, unpleasant smell familiar to the patient but which he *cannot* name is a common manifestation of a temporal lobe seizure.

The pathways subserving the sense of smell, paleobiologically one of our most important protective sensory systems, have no apparent thalamic connections. **Central anosmia** does not exist, although anosmia is marked in demented patients.

The patient with fictitious anosmia can sometimes be identified with ammonia. It irritates the nose, causes tearing, and stops respiration. The irritation is transmitted via the fifth cranial nerve. Test results for the other functions of the fifth cranial nerve are normal. The patient says he cannot tell the difference between ammonia and tap water when they are consecutively placed under his nose. This is not consistent with organic disease.

FIFTH CRANIAL NERVE

The fifth cranial (trigeminal) nerve is a mixed nerve. It contains motor and sensory fibers. Most of the diseases of this nerve and its connections are disturbances of **sensation**. Motor lesions are relatively rare.

Peripheral Anatomy

The first division, or ophthalmic branch, leaves the cranial vault through the **superior orbital fissure** and surfaces onto the face through the **superior orbital foramen**. Read again the sections on lesions of the third, fourth, and sixth cranial nerves (Chapter 4) in the cavernous sinus and at the superior orbital fissure; you will find most of the lesions of this division of the trigeminal nerve. This division supplies the area labeled "1" in Figure 8–1—the cornea, the mucous membrane of the upper nose, and some meninges.

The second division, or maxillary branch, leaves the cranial vault through the foramen rotundum and surfaces through the infra-orbital foramen. This division supplies the area labeled "2" in Figure 8–1—the mucous membrane of the lower nose, the upper jaw, upper teeth, and anterior palate.

The third division, or mandibular branch, leaves the cranial vault through the foramen ovale and surfaces through the mental foramen. This division is also *motor* to the **pterygoids, masseter, temporalis, mylohyoid,** and anterior belly of the **digastric muscles**. This division supplies (sensory) area 3 in Figure 8–1—the tongue, the lower teeth, and the mucous membrane of the floor of the mouth, cheek, and lower lip.

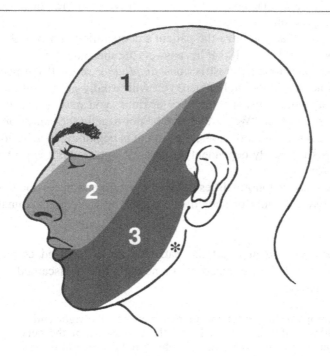

Figure 8–1. The three cutaneous sensory divisions of the trigeminal nerve. The area marked with an asterisk is not part of the trigeminal nerve and is part of the territory of the greater auricular nerve (C2 and C3).

There is *no* overlap between the areas supplied by the three peripheral divisions of the trigeminal nerve, unlike the situation with the spinal nerves. All three divisions supply sensation to the dura.

Sensory Testing

All sensory deficits are subjective. There are reflexes, conduction velocities, and evoked responses that can assess sensory function with variable sensitivity and objectivity. However, most of our information about the patient's sensory systems is obtained at the bedside or in the office with a pin, a tuning fork, a wisp of cotton wool, and a few other crude instruments. Only the patient can judge the quality of what he feels. You must stay out of the decision; that is, if you are testing his response to pinprick on the right and left sides of the face, you may obtain one answer by saying to him, "Is this [touching the pin to the right] the *same* as this [touching the left]?," and a completely different answer by saying (under the same circumstances), "Is this . . . *different* from this . . . ?" You will have planted the word *different* or *same* in the patient's mind. Most patients are helpful and agreeable and may honestly think that one side is less sensitive than the other because of the way the question was asked.

It is essential that you have the patient's cooperation and confidence, and he must not be tired or so ill that his answers are meaningless.

Keep your questions and instructions *simple and short*. If the patient is a child or an adult of low intelligence, you will usually get a short, definitive answer. From others, usually the very anxious, you may get an overinterpreted answer, such as "Well . . . , maybe not exactly the same" or "Would you do that again?" In these cases, the patient is beginning to alert you that if this diagnosis is heavily dependent on sensory signs only, it is probably going to be wrong.

Complex sensory abnormalities deserve an examination session devoted to the sensory system only or should be verified by a repeat examination the next day.

Pain Perception Do not hurt the patient. Use a sterilized common pin. Each patient should be examined with a new pin that is discarded at the end of the examination.

> Compare the perception of pain between the right and left sides in the first, second, and third divisions of the nerve; that is, touch the patient's forehead lightly several times on the right side with the pin. Do the same on the left, asking the patient whether they feel the same. Then compare the right cheek with the left cheek and the right chin with the left chin.

Apply the same procedure for touch.

> Have the patient close her eyes and, using the wisp of cotton
> wool, ask her to say "yes" each time you touch her.

Do not drag the cotton wisp over the skin: this is tickling, which is allied to pain. A touch is an end-point contact. Some touches may be normally ignored. Does the patient feel the same number of touches on the right side of the face as on the left when her eyes are closed? The central connections for touch and pain are different. Thus, the loss of one sensation and preservation of the other in the same part of the face may help to localize the lesion.

Corneal Reflex The cornea is sensitive to pain. The response to corneal stimulation is *bilateral* blinking.

> Ask the patient to look straight ahead; touch the cornea with
> a rolled-up piece of tissue or cotton wool.

Figure 8–2 shows three common mistakes in eliciting the corneal reflex: (a) The stimulus is touching the eyelash. This will always provoke a blink, so you do not know whether the corneal reflex is present. (b) The stimulus is touching the sclera. This is less sensitive than the cornea and is not the area from which the reflex initiates. (c) The stimulus is in front of the pupil, so

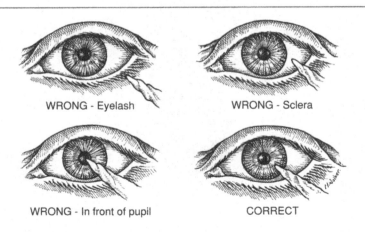

Figure 8–2. Three common errors in eliciting the corneal reflex. The stimulus touches the eyelash or the sclera or is in front of the pupil. In the lower right it is placed correctly on the cornea.

the patient can see it coming. He can hardly resist blinking, whether or not the cornea is touched. The final frame in Figure 8–2 shows the stimulus touching the cornea correctly.

If the patient will not let you touch his cornea, ask him to look *up* and to the *left* when you test his right corneal reflex (Figure 8–3). It is then quite simple to touch his cornea from below without startling him. To test the left cornea, have him look up and to the right.

You may have trouble with the fluttering eyelids of the patient who cannot let anything come near his eye. Ask him to forcefully open his mouth as *wide* as he can. This will give you a 5- to 10-s blink-free period to test his corneal reflexes. It will not work repeatedly or for very long, so be ready to do the reflex and then ask the patient to open his mouth.

The corneal reflex

- Will often vanish with lesions of the **first division** or **root** before you can demonstrate any sensory disturbance of touch, pain, or temperature sensation in area 1 of Figure 8–1
- Is absent when contact lenses cover the cornea. These now fit so well and precisely over the cornea that they are difficult to see.

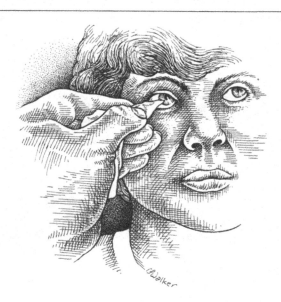

Figure 8–3. It is helpful when testing the patient's right corneal reflex to have her look up and to the left and bring the stimulus in from below and from the right.

- Is often absent after cataract surgery
- Is often absent in elderly people, for unknown reasons
- Has a supranuclear connection to the opposite thalamus. In acute destructive lesions (hemorrhage) into the thalamus, the contralateral corneal reflex will be *absent* and then present but delayed for days or a week or so after the ictus. Superficial hemisphere lesions do not do this.

The Spinal Nucleus and the Tract of the Trigeminal Nerve

The spinal nucleus and tract of the trigeminal nerve

- Extends from the midpons at the level of entry of the trigeminal root to the upper cervical spinal segments
- Blends into and is continuous with the substantia gelatinosa of the cervical cord
- Subserves the functions of pain and temperature sensation, touch being a function of the **main sensory nucleus**, which is at the rostral end of the spinal nucleus

Fibers from the ophthalmic division of the nerve are most ventral in the tract and those from the mandibular division are most dorsal, with the maxillary fibers in the middle.

The spinal trigeminal nucleus is *medial* to the tract and divided into three areas corresponding to the areas shown in Figure 8–4 at A, B, and C. These areas do not have the same cutaneous relationships as the three peripheral branches. Area A cuts through all three peripheral divisions and has its cellular components in the most rostral part of the nucleus, area B is intermediate, and area C is related to the most caudal end of the nucleus. (For an excellent account of the anatomy of the nucleus, see A. Brodal, *Neurological Anatomy in Relation to Clinical Medicine*, 3rd ed. Oxford University Press, New York, 1981, p. 528.)

When pain loss involves parts of all three peripheral divisions of the trigeminal nerve, consider the possibility of a **nuclear location** of the lesion.

Temperature Sensation

Hot and cold sensations are not commonly examined on the face. However, it may be a useful thing to do. When a patient complains of pain or numbness in the face and the conventional pain-touch sensory examination as outlined above reveals no abnormalities, there may be some decreased awareness of temperature differences over the face. This can precede the loss of pain. Temperature sensation should not be examined as a routine measure (see the section on "Temperature" in Chapter 14).

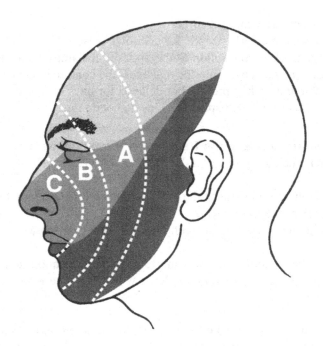

Figure 8–4. The cutaneous representation of pain perception by the three divisions of the spinal trigeminal nucleus. Area C has its cellular components in the rostral part of the nucleus and area A is in the caudal part of the nucleus, while area B is intermediate.

Motor Function

The motor function of the fifth cranial nerve is mediated through the **mandibular**, or third, division. In the presence of a fifth nerve lesion there will be paralysis and atrophy of the temporalis, masseter, and pterygoid muscles. When the mouth is opened, the mandible deviates *toward the paralyzed side*.

- Watch the patient open his mouth several times, and pay particular attention to the direction the mandible takes as the mouth opens.
- Put the tips of your index fingers along the most anterior edges of the patient's masseter muscles.
- Do this with the patient's mouth closed but his jaw relaxed.
- Ask him to bite firmly.

Your fingers will move forward as indicated in Figure 8–5. If one masseter is weaker or smaller than the other, it will be obvious in the relative lack of movement of your finger.

The absence of teeth on one side and a defective or faulty bite may eventually result in a reduced masseter bulk.

Similarly, you can get more information by feeling the temporalis contracting than by looking at it.

Diseases of the Fifth Nerve

Pain in the Face Possible causes include

- Carotid artery aneurysm (reread the sections on the third, fourth, and sixth cranial nerves in Chapter 4)
- Carcinoma nasopharynx

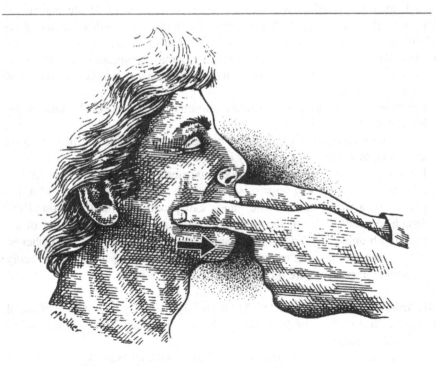

Figure 8–5. To feel the masseter muscles contract, place your fingers in *front* of the *edge* of the muscle as the patient bites down firmly. Your fingers will move forward (arrow).

- Raeder's paratrigeminal neuralgia
- Metastases to the base of the skull
- Herpes zoster
- Cluster headaches
- Angina pectoris
- Tic douloureux, or short, sharp, excruciating pain that travels in the anatomical distribution of one or sometimes two cutaneous divisions of the nerve. The mandibular division is most common. Pain lasts for seconds, with 20–200 stabs per day, precipitated by talking, eating, drinking, washing the face, or exposure to cold air. There is often a precise trigger point; touching it invariably initiates pain. It is most common in middle and late life, although it also occurs in younger people as a manifestation of multiple sclerosis.

Numbness (Analgesia, Hyperesthesia, or Paresthesia) in the Face Causes include

- Lesions in the cerebellar pontine angle, for example, acoustic neuroma—as it grows upward, it will elevate and stretch the root of the trigeminal nerve before the latter perforates the tentorium. There will be signs of involvement of the seventh (late) and eighth (early) cranial nerves.
- Multiple sclerosis, brain stem infarct, glioma, syringobulbia, and some medications, for example, streptomycin, pyridoxine, isoniazid, and some kinds of penicillin
- Fractures or metastatic and primary tumors of the bones of the face or the base of the skull
- Trigeminal neuropathy of unknown cause, usually in women. It is progressive, bilateral, and will eventually involve the entire face.
- **Bilateral**, circumoral numbness does *not* mean the patient necessarily has a bilateral lesion. Focal sensory seizures, the somatic paresthesias of a migraine, or a transient ischemic attack can produce numbness around the mouth, on *both* sides of the midline. The secondary representation of *all* the mouth and lips (and tongue) is in both the right and left hemispheres. (The trigeminothalamic tracts subserving touch and pressure and probably pain and temperature are *both* crossed and uncrossed.)

Weakness of Jaw Movements Myotonic dystrophy will produce bilateral weakness and wasting of both temporalis and masseters although jaw opening muscles seem strong.

Myasthenia gravis will produce weakness without wasting of both jaw openers and closers.

Amyotrophic lateral sclerosis and poliomyelitis also cause weakness and wasting of both jaw openers and closers.

Unilateral—fracture or neoplasm or inflammation of the foramen ovale; the jaw is *pulled* over to the *paretic* side by the *pterygoids* of the normal side (PPP).

In a *unilateral* upper motor neuron lesion, jaw opening and closing is normal. Both hemispheres innervate both right and left muscles that open and close the jaw.

- **Bilateral** upper motor neuron lesions produce an abnormality of chewing that is part of pseudobulbar palsy (described in Chapter 16).

SEVENTH CRANIAL NERVE

The seventh cranial (facial) nerve is a great nerve—with it we can laugh, frown, cry, taste, and spit!

Anatomy

The seventh nerve is an important **mixed** nerve with motor, sensory, and autonomic divisions.

Motor Function

The motor fibers supply the muscles of facial expression, from frontalis to platysma, the stapedius muscle in the middle ear, the stylohyoid, and the posterior belly of the digastric. A lesion of the nerve trunk or its nucleus produces a lower motor neuron palsy and is described as a seventh nerve lesion. It affects *all* the muscles partially or completely supplied by the nerve. By contrast, facial weakness caused by a contralateral **upper motor neuron lesion** presents a distinctly different clinical picture.

The terms *seventh nerve lesion* and *facial weakness* are not interchangeable. The first means an ipsilateral lesion of the lower motor neuron and paralysis of all the muscles of one side of the face. The latter means a contralateral lesion of the upper motor neuron and variable weakness of some of the muscles of one side of the face.

Remember:

- The frontalis muscle is supplied by the ipsilateral and contralateral hemispheres. In facial weakness (the upper motor neuron lesion) the forehead on the side of the weakness *appears* to wrinkle in a normal way. If you ask the patient to wrinkle upward against resistance, you can *feel* a slight weakness on the abnormal side relative to the normal. In a seventh nerve lesion the ipsilateral forehead is flat and will not wrinkle at all.
- The orbicularis oculi also have bilateral suprasegmental innervation. With the upper motor neuron lesion causing facial weakness, the eye will close

but is weaker than the normal side and the difference is easy to detect with your fingers. With the seventh nerve lesion the eye will not close at all and is open *wider* on the paretic side.

How to Examine the Seventh Cranial Nerve

1. **Look at the patient when she is at rest and while she is talking, smiling, and blinking.**
2. **Ask her to wrinkle her forehead quickly two or three times (the Groucho Marx maneuver) (Figure 8–6A). Watch the rate and extent of the movement of the two eyebrows. When the patient is relaxed, put your finger on her eyebrows and ask her to wrinkle her forehead against this gentle resistance.**
3. **Ask her to close her eyes gently, then tightly (Figure 8–6B). Try to open them while the patient resists you.** If she can wrinkle her forehead and can close her eyes, this is not a seventh nerve lesion.
4. **Now compare the lower right side of the face with the left side and look for *relative* weakness on one side, as in facial weakness resulting from an upper motor neuron lesion. Ask the patient to close her eyes as tightly as she can.** Did the patient
   - Tuck in the eyelashes between the edges of the lids equally well right and left? They will *not* tuck in as far on the side of a facial weakness.
   - Deepen the nasolabial groove equally well right and left? It will *not* deepen as much on the side of a facial weakness.
   - Retract the corners of her mouth away from the midline *equally far* right and left? The corner of the mouth on the side of a facial weakness will not move as far (Figure 8–6B).
5. **Ask the patient to show her teeth.** (The occasional patient with dentures will hand them to you at this point; everyone else with dentures will tell you their teeth are not their own.) Ask the patient to clench her teeth together and retract the corners of her mouth. Again, notice whether the two corners go equally far and equally fast. Sometimes the only manifestation of a facial weakness is the momentary delay by one corner of the mouth, which begins to move 1 s later than on the normal side.
6. **Ask the patient to whistle. Ask her to press her lips together and blow up her cheeks; tap on one and then the other inflated cheek.** Air will escape between the lips when you tap the weak side (Figure 8–6C).
7. **Ask the patient to open her mouth as wide as she can.** The opening should be symmetrical, with the same number of teeth showing on the two sides of the midline. The weak side of the face covers *more* teeth than the normal side.

To see the patient's platysma, you have to act as a model (Figure 8–6D). Do the following, by way of example, then ask her to repeat your actions.

8. **Clench your teeth and pull the corners of your mouth forcefully downward with a grimace, revealing your platysma.**

At rest, the patient with a **seventh nerve lesion** has, on the *paretic side*,

- An eye open *wider* than on the normal side; it does not blink; increased tears are stimulated by the dry and irritated cornea and flow over the paretic cheek.
- A flat, creaseless forehead
- A flat, sometimes drooping cheek
- The corner of the mouth lower than on the normal side
- A "flappy," loose cheek as he talks
- The midsagittal line of the mouth pulled over to the normal side

At rest, the patient with a **facial weakness** may *look* perfectly normal or show a minor flattening and asymmetry.

Remember that normal elderly people may have an asymmetrical lower face at rest. This is because of an asymmetrical loss of teeth, a lifetime habit of talking out of the corner of the mouth, or simple passage of time. (Look carefully at the next 12 people over 65 years of age that you meet. Most of them have some asymmetry about the mouth and difference in the depth of the two nasolabial folds.)

The patient with a seventh nerve lesion is equally unable to perform voluntary, reflex, or emotional movements of half of the face.

In contrast, the patient with a facial weakness has paresis and slowness, mostly of the lower half of the face, for voluntary movements but smiling is normal and symmetrical. If you can make him laugh, the paretic side of the face seems to move as well or more than the normal side. Why? Either emotional facial movements have bilateral supranuclear connections (which is probably correct) or the upper motor neuron for voluntary movements is completely different from the supranuclear fibers concerned with smiling, frowning, laughing, and crying. A patient with a **hemifacial defect** for emotional movements only, but a normal face for voluntary movements and a solitary lesion in the opposite thalamus, has been described (See N Engl J Med 1998; 338(21):1515).

Blinking

Watch the patient blink. If he blinks less often than you do, he may have parkinsonism or may be abusing some sedative. The eyes blink at exactly the same moment and the eye is completely covered with each blink. If he

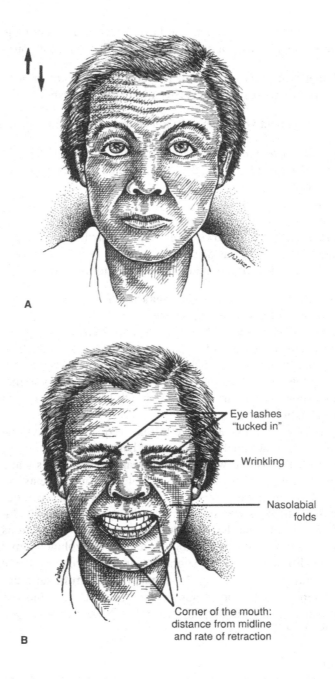

Figure 8–6. A. Testing the frontalis muscle and seventh nerve function by asking the patient to repeatedly wrinkle and relax the forehead in the direction of the arrows. **B.** Forceful eye closing reveals the symmetry of eyelash tucking, wrinkling around the eyes, depth of the nasolabial folds, and retraction of the corners of the mouth. (*Continued*)

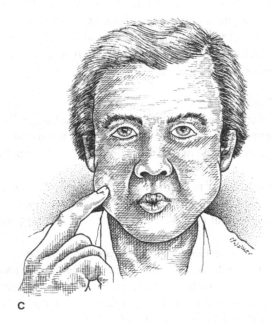

C

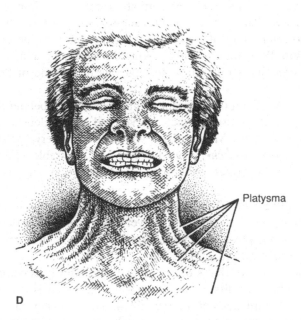

Platysma

D

Figure 8–6 (continued). C. The patient purses his lips together and distends his cheeks by blowing into them. Tap one cheek and then the other. Air will escape between the lips on the weak side. **D.** Clenching the teeth and forcefully pulling the corners of the mouth downward reveals the symmetry of mouth movement and the platysma.

blinks less often on the right side or does not cover the entire right eye with each blink, he has a partial right seventh nerve lesion, new or old. This is never the result of an upper motor neuron facial weakness or a fifth cranial nerve lesion. Asynchronous blinking is most often seen in the patient with a partially recovered Bell's palsy.

Sensory and Autonomic

The **intermediate nerve** or **sensory root** of cranial nerve 7 emerges from the brain stem between the facial motor root and the vestibular (eighth) nerve. If it had its own cranial nerve number, it would be $7^1/2$. Its functions are

- Taste—From the anterior two thirds of the tongue, cells are in the **geniculate ganglion**, and central termination is on the rostral part of the **solitary nucleus**. The peripheral pathway is via the chorda tympani and lingual nerves.
- Saliva—The cells are in the dorsolateral reticular formation, called the **superior salivatory nucleus**. Fibers that are preganglionic and parasympathetic travel in the intermediate nerve, then in the chorda tympani and lingual nerves to the **submandibular ganglion**. Postganglionic fibers go to the submandibular and sublingual salivary glands.
- Tears—Have the same reticular formation cells of origin as described above for saliva. Parasympathetic preganglionic fibers leave the intermediate nerve to enter the greater superficial petrosal nerve to the **pterygopalatine ganglion**. Postganglionic fibers go to the lacrimal gland, and secretory and vasomotor fibers proceed to the mucous membrane of the nose and mouth.
- Pain fibers—Are from the external auditory canal and behind the ear. The fibers are part of the intermediate nerve, and the nucleus is part of the spinal trigeminal tract. Most patients with a seventh nerve palsy complain of numbness over the *cheek* but have no demonstrable sensory loss to touch, pain, or temperature examination on the cheek or anywhere else.

Taste, Tears, and Saliva Taste from the anterior two thirds of the tongue is an *afferent* function of the seventh nerve. Taste from the posterior tongue and palate is via the **glossopharyngeal nerve**, which is more important than the seventh nerve in this function.

From the anterior two thirds of the tongue the pathway is complex as follows: (a) the fibers are first in the lingual nerve, which is a branch of the mandibular (the third division of the trigeminal); (b) they are then in the chorda tympani nerve (a branch of cranial nerve 7) to their cell station, which is the geniculate ganglion; and (c) from here are in the intermediate nerve, which is the sensory root of the seventh cranial nerve.

Centrally, the fibers connect with the nucleus of the solitary tract and probably to both ipsilateral and contralateral thalamus and sensory cortex.

How to Test Taste

1. **Ask the patient to protrude his tongue. Place the dorsal surface of your left index finger horizontally against his chin. Hold a tissue draped over your index finger. When the tongue comes out over your finger, grasp it between your index finger and thumb, using the tissue to improve your grip (Figure 8–7). Tell the patient not to try to answer but to hold up his hand if he tastes something.**
2. **Use a slightly damp applicator stick dipped in granulated sugar or salt as a test substance.** These are better in the dry form rather than in solution. Liquids may flow over the tongue and you then would not know which side you are testing.

Tastes can be identified by most patients in about 3–10 s. Do not release the tongue. With another applicator stick covered with the same substance, stroke the other side of the tongue and time this. You may find that taste is perceived on one side after 5 s and after 30 s or not at all on the other side.

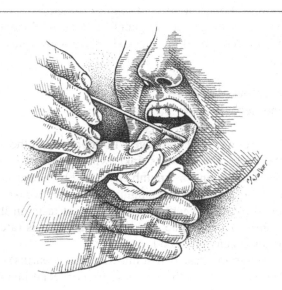

Figure 8–7. To test taste, hold the tongue as shown and apply the test substance with the applicator stick.

The slow side is the abnormal one. As soon as you let go of the tongue the examination is over. The sugar is then tasted from many areas inside the mouth. The test can be repeated after 5 min and after the patient has rinsed his mouth.

Remember:

- There is not much taste sense on the tip of the tongue.
- Elderly people lose their sense of taste and the number of taste buds.
- Some people cannot perceive sugar on either side of the tongue. Allow such a patient to rinse out his mouth and try a different substance.
- In general, taste is perceived better on the more posterior aspects of the tongue, palate, and pharynx rather than on the anterior.
- There are only four taste substances: sweet, sour (acid), bitter (quinine), and salty.
- A lesion of the seventh nerve at the stylomastoid foramen where it emerges from the skull (commonly caused by trauma or disease of the parotid gland) produces a seventh nerve lesion as described above, with no taste loss and no hyperacusis.
- A lesion distal to the geniculate ganglion (Bell's palsy being the most common) produces the paresis as above, loss of taste in the anterior two thirds of the tongue, hyperacusis (the branch to the stapedius), and a decrease of salivary secretion on the same side. (Review the anatomy of the intermediate nerve mentioned briefly at the start of this chapter.)
- A lesion proximal to the geniculate ganglion (a cerebellopontile angle tumor being the most common) produces all of the above plus a dry eye on the same side.

Diseases of the Seventh Nerve

Diseases of this nerve include

- Bell's palsy—Onset may be at any age with **pain** behind the ear and down the side of the neck. The cause is unknown. The lesion is in the facial canal; the patient complains of a numb cheek and hyperacusis on the same side, as well as facial paralysis. Examination reveals weakness of all the muscles supplied by the seventh nerve and absent taste on the ipsilateral anterior two thirds of the tongue. It can be bilateral, it is rarely recurrent, and the prognosis is generally good.
- Guillain-Barré syndrome (also called infectious polyneuritis)—Often bilateral, it may start with a seventh nerve lesion(s) or facial involvement may occur after the arms and legs are involved.
- Sarcoidosis, vasculitis, parotid gland tumor, leprosy, infectious mononucleosis, and Lyme disease

- Acute or chronic otitis media and mastoiditis
- The cerebellar-pontine angle tumor—Seventh nerve palsy signs are both rare and late and generally follow the deafness and trigeminal nerve signs and symptoms. The ipsilateral eye will not tear.
- Geniculate ganglion herpes—Herpes zoster in the external ear canal, concha, and mouth and behind the ear; pain in the ear; paralysis of the face as in Bell's palsy with the same taste loss. Herpes, pain, and facial weakness may all appear at once or consecutively over several days. Taste recovery is unlikely.
- Within the pons—Vascular disease, poliomyelitis, neoplasm demyelinating lesions, and syringobulbia

Bilateral Seventh Nerve Palsy

- Bell's palsy
- Guillain-Barré syndrome
- Encephalitis
- Prepontine, intrapontine tumor
- Meningitis, cryptococcal or tuberculous, and as part of acquired immune deficiency
- Sarcoid, systemic lupus erythematosus

Diseases Causing Facial Weakness

Any lesions that occur in the internal capsule or any other part of the upper motor neuron above the seventh nerve nucleus (eg, vascular lesion, neoplasm, abscess, or trauma) can produce an upper motor neuron facial weakness.

Parkinsonism Parkinsonism can be exclusively unilateral or at least much more marked in one arm and leg, but if the face is involved it is always on both sides. The patient can wrinkle his forehead, close his eyes, show his teeth, whistle, and so on, so clearly the face is not paretic. However, the emotional responses revealed by the face are absent. A hemifacial defect for emotional expression can occur from a lesion in the contralateral thalamus (see page 99).

Cranial Nerves 8–12

9

EIGHTH NERVE

The eighth (acoustic) nerve is really two nerves—the cochlear (meaning "snail shell"), which is concerned with hearing, and the vestibular (meaning "cavity at a canal entrance"), which is concerned with movement, position, and balance.

Cochlear Nerve

Lesions of this special sensory nerve cause deafness. Nerve cells are in the spiral ganglion of the cochlea. Their peripheral connections are to the auditory cells of the **organ of Corti**, and their central connections are to the **cochlear nucleus**. The next-order neuron is the lateral lemniscus. When impulses concerned with sound have reached the cochlear nucleus, their further passage is bilateral (ie, a unilateral lesion above the level of the nucleus cannot cause deafness).

Deafness Does the patient have some hearing loss, and if so, is it nerve deafness (or sensorineural deafness) or conductive deafness? Conductive deafness is caused by a disease of the external canal, middle ear, or ossicles. The key features of nerve deafness are

- Loss of perception of *high pitched* sounds
- Loss of hearing of *bone conducted* sound

How to Examine Hearing You can learn a lot from the patient's history. If the patient can hear on the telephone using either ear, his hearing is reasonably good.

A formal test is awareness of whispered speech at 6 ft. It is often difficult to find a quiet room in which to test the patient. Follow this method:

- Have the patient stand, facing at right angles to you, at a distance of 6 ft.
- Ask the patient to put his finger in the ear farther from you. Whisper a series of numbers, asking him to repeat each number after you.

A person with normal hearing can hear and repeat nine out of 10 whispered numbers at this distance. Then turn the patient so that he faces the opposite way, ask him to plug the far ear, and repeat the procedure. Your whispered voice can vary from very faint to almost conversational speech. After you have done this a few times, you will get the sense of a constant-volume whisper and the test becomes quite reliable. If his hearing is normal, record it as "Whispered voice @ 6′, Rt and Lt." If you had to move up for the patient to hear the numbers when testing the left ear, record it as, for example, "Whispered voice @ 6′ Rt and 4′ Lt."

If the patient is deaf in one or both ears, do the following to establish whether the deafness is caused by a defect in the conducting system of the ear or in the nerve leading from the ear.

- Place the handle of a vibrating 256 tuning fork on the patient's mastoid.
- Ask him to tell you when the vibrations can no longer be heard.
- At that point, put the vibrating tines of the tuning fork close to the patient's ear.

If the sound reappears, one can say that *air conduction is better than bone conduction*. These are the findings in most people *and* in **early nerve deafness**. If *your* hearing is normal, put the handle of the 256 tuning fork on the patient's mastoid and when he says he can no longer hear it, put the handle on your own mastoid. If you hear it through your mastoid longer than the patient does, he has nerve deafness. If nerve deafness is complete, there is no appreciation of sound by either bone conduction or air conduction. This is the **Rinne test**. It is reliable only with bilateral hearing loss. The opposite situation—when bone conduction is longer than air conduction—is found in conductive or middle ear deafness.

There is another way to tell nerve deafness from conductive deafness:

Put the handle of a vibrating 256 tuning fork on the center of the patient's head, over the vertex. Ask him if he hears it better in one ear or the other or in the center of his head.

If the patient has a conductive hearing loss in one ear, he will hear the tuning fork in this ear. You can simulate this for yourself, provided that you have normal hearing. When the vibrating tuning fork is on the vertex of your head, put your finger in one ear. The sound will immediately become loudest in this ear. You have thus produced a degree of conductive deafness in yourself. This is the **Weber test**. On the other hand, if the patient has nerve deafness in one ear, he will hear the tuning fork in the opposite normal ear. Weber's test is no help in bilateral deafness and it will not work if there is both nerve and conductive deafness in the same ear.

Remember, **nerve deafness** results in decreased bone conduction and loss of high-tone appreciation; **conduction deafness** results in decreased air conduction and loss of low-tone appreciation. Total hearing loss always means nerve deafness.

Vestibular Nerve

Test the vestibular nerve and vestibular apparatus (the semicircular canals, utricle, and saccule) by observing the movements and position of the eyes. This also assesses the function of the brain stem from the upper medulla to the midbrain.

The patient with an acute unilateral vestibular lesion has vertigo and vomiting and staggers to the side of the lesion. The vertigo is spinning of the environment (object vertigo) to the opposite side. Her eyes are forced to the side of the lesion, and she has nystagmus to the opposite side, that is, the fast component. A chronic or slowly progressive lesion of the semicircular canals or the vestibular nerve will likely have none of these signs and symptoms.

How to Test Vestibular Function The otologists and clinical neurophysiologists have sophisticated ways of testing the function of both divisions of the eighth cranial nerve. At the bedside the principal testing method is observation of eye movements in response to hot and cold water in the external ear canal, that is, **caloric testing.** Cold water inhibits the function of the semicircular canals, whereas warm water enhances it. If a temporary imbalance can be created between the two sides, the system can be tested. Cold-water stimulation of the external ear canal simulates acute destructive labyrinthine disease, that is, eyes to the irrigated side, nystagmus away from the irrigated side. A mnemonic in Joel S. Glaser's *Neurophthalmology* (Harper & Row, Hagerstown, Maryland, 1978) will help you remember the nystagmus direction:

COWS: Cold–Opposite–Warm–Same

- Sit the patient with her head in extension, occiput supported, looking at the ceiling, or have her lie on her back with her head on a pillow 30 degrees from the horizontal. Her horizontal semicircular canal is now vertical.
- Look in the external ear with an otoscope. Remove any wax in the external canal. If the tympanic membrane is perforated or red and bulging, **stop now**.
- Put a large kidney basin under the ear, with the concave side against the neck. Put a folded towel under the basin, and *slowly and gently* inject 20 mL of cold (20°C) tap water over 20–30 s.

• Time the onset, duration, and direction of nystagmus. Wait 10 min and do the same to the other ear (check first for wax, perforation, and so on).

The interval and duration should be approximately the same, right and left, as should the degree of discomfort, nausea, spinning sensation, or vomiting.

• Repeat the irrigations after an interval using warm (42°C) water in first one and then the other ear.

If a patient has just recovered from an episode that you suspect was acute labyrinthitis or has had chronic recurrent episodes of vertigo, ataxia, vomiting, or dizziness, try *warm* water first. Cold-water irrigation in such patients is often less effective.

Vestibular Function in the Unconscious Patient Reread the section on "The Doll's Eye Test and Caloric Testing" in Chapter 7.

Use water as cold as you can find. This is a stronger stimulus than the hottest tolerable hot water. The purpose of the examination has changed. This is an attempt to *localize* the lesion responsible for the coma.

The full ocular deviation to one side and nystagmus to the other test the integrity of the vestibular nerve, nuclei, medial longitudinal fasciculus, oculomotor nuclei, brain stem reticular mechanisms, and hemispheres.

• When the cause of the coma is a pontine lesion, the response is *absent*. Be careful! If the patient's coma is because he is frozen or drug-overloaded, this false absent response is reversible. If in doubt, repeat the examination in 12 and 24 hr.
• If the response is *normal* (remember in the unconscious patient there is no nystagmus, and *normal* means eye deviation only), the cause of the coma is not in the brain stem.
• If the response is only *abduction* of one eye, the cause of the coma is in the midbrain. The oculomotor nuclear constellation is damaged, and adduction cannot occur.

Diseases of the Eighth Cranial Nerve

When the patient has vertigo, tinnitus, and deafness, the diagnostic possibilities are many. As always, start with a careful history. Vertigo can be postural in the arteriosclerotic elderly patient and in others who are on tricyclic antidepressant drugs. It can also be part of the symptom complex of a temporal lobe seizure or can be perfectly benign in the long-legged male youth who seems to be growing like a weed and says that every time he stands up quickly the room spins and his vision fades, and he has actually fallen twice in the past 6 months.

Deafness must be differentiated as to nerve, conduction, or mixed, and the lesion may result from an acoustic neuroma, presbyacusis, otosclerosis, Meniere's disease, chronic ear infection, industrial abuse, trauma, or drugs (eg, kanamycin).

Tinnitus Tinnitus is described as a ringing, whistling, buzzing, clicking, or roaring in the ears. It may be present in one or both ears and can sometimes even be heard by persons other than the patient.

Tinnitus is a common complaint and is a symptom rarely relieved. It is thought to be peripheral (nerve or more distal) in origin, but there may be central causes.

Tinnitus can be present early with an acoustic neuroma. By the time the patient is deaf and seeks help, months or years may have passed, and he is no longer aware of the tinnitus. Some patients with Meniere's disease seem to be able to forget their violent attacks of vertigo, tinnitus, and vomiting and will go to the doctor years later because of progressing deafness.

Aspirin causes and aggravates tinnitus, but some patients never make the connection. The sound may be rushing or pulsating and is always louder at night in the quiet of the bedroom. You may hear the patient's noise with your stethoscope. If the patient is elderly and invasive investigations would be hazardous, avoid such procedures.

Occasionally, a patient with increased intracranial pressure complains of a pulsating sound in her head that other members of the family can also hear. Some vessel in the head is being compressed. The sound vanishes when the pressure is reduced.

When a patient sleeps on her side, she may compress the occipital branch of the posterior auricular artery between the skull and the pillow. This can produce a pulsating, swishing sound. This is harmless.

NINTH NERVE

The ninth (glossopharyngeal) nerve is both sensory and motor. Its only motor function is to the stylopharyngeus muscle. This cannot be tested clinically. The nerve supplies sensation to the tympanic cavity, the tonsils, the posterior aspect of the soft palate (as does the maxillary branch of the trigeminal nerve), the posterior third of the tongue, and the pharynx. It carries taste fibers from the posterior third of the tongue and supplies secretory fibers to the parotid gland.

How to Examine the Glossopharyngeal Nerve Sensation on the pharynx can be tested with an applicator stick that has no cotton on it.

- Compare the response of the right and left halves of the pharynx by touching them gently with the end of the stick.
- You can ask the patient whether touching the pharynx feels the same right and left, and you may provoke a gag reflex on one side, but not the other.

The motor side of this reflex is a prompt contraction of the pharynx with or without gagging. In many people pharyngeal contraction and gagging cannot be elicited from either side. Abnormalities of palatal and pharyngeal sensation are soft physical signs, and there is not a high diagnostic yield in this part of the examination. You cannot test the taste on the posterior part of the tongue.

Diseases of the ninth and tenth cranial nerves are considered together after the section on the tenth nerve.

TENTH NERVE

The tenth (vagus) nerve is also a mixed nerve. It has afferent fibers from the dura of the posterior fossa, the external ear, pharynx, larynx, trachea, esophagus, and thoracic and abdominal viscera. It sends parasympathetic fibers to the thoracic and abdominal viscera and motor fibers to the muscles of the palate, pharynx, and larynx. Review the anatomy of the vagus, with attention to the superior laryngeal nerve and the two recurrent laryngeal nerves.

The neurological examination of the vagus concerns mostly the muscles of the palate, the constrictors and sphincter of the pharynx, and the muscles of the larynx.

Palate

In the palate there may be no symptoms from unilateral paresis. However, on examination the arch on the paretic side is lower.

Ask the patient to quickly say "ah."

The midline of the palate will go over to the normal side, the normal arch will lift and curve, and the paretic side will remain lower and straighten (Figure 9–1A and B). The uvula is not important. It is soft and floppy and sometimes hangs in the midline or to the right or left. Ignore it.

Bilateral palatal paralysis causes nasal regurgitation and a nasal voice, and it is difficult for the patient to pronounce *b* and *g*. You can *hear* air coming out of his nose as he talks.

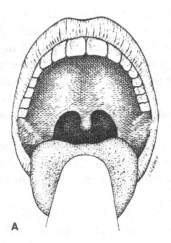 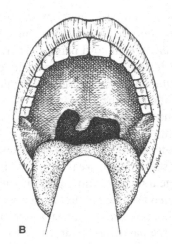

Figure 9–1. A. Normal palatal arches. **B.** Paretic left arch. As the patient says "ah," the midline shifts to the right and the right arch rises and curves, while the left remains lower and straight.

The gag reflex was described with the glossopharyngeal nerve. Many people normally have no gag reflex, while others will start gagging as soon as you put a tongue blade on the tongue and before you have touched the palate or pharynx. There is physiological testing of the gag reflex every time the patient swallows. If he can manage liquids without nasal regurgitation, his palate lifts.

Pharynx

The constrictor muscles of the pharynx cause the food bolus to "turn the corner" out of the mouth and then force it into the esophagus. A patient with paresis of the pharynx will tell you that, in spite of lengthy chewing, the food will not go down. She also has bubbling speech because mucus and saliva (and food) remain in the pharynx and overflow into the larynx. This causes coughing. Such patients repeatedly clear the throat with poor results. The gag reflex is absent. Unilateral pharyngeal paresis is tolerable, with minimal or moderate dysphagia, coughing, and a bubbly voice. Bilateral pharyngeal paresis is a disaster of coughing, choking, and dysphagia. Every attempted meal is a trial, and a full night's sleep is an impossibility.

Larynx

Unilateral paresis of the larynx can produce a hoarse, weak voice that improves with time as the opposite normal cord crosses the midline. Even if the patient, his family, and you think his voice is *normal*, he may still have a *unilateral* vocal cord paresis. There is often trouble with swallowing liquids if the lesion is peripheral and involves the recurrent laryngeal nerve only. Both the abductor and adductor muscles of the larynx *and* the lower sphincter of the pharynx are paretic.

If the lesion is more proximal, palatal and pharyngeal paresis will also be present.

Bilateral paresis with a distal lesion (thyroidectomy) presents as a stridulous (see stridor), weak voice with shortness of breath. The intact superior laryngeal nerve (a more proximal branch of the vagus nerve) keeps the cords adducted and the airway dangerously narrow.

With more proximal lesions causing bilateral paresis, there is usually paresis of the palate and pharynx as well. The vocal cords are in midposition, the voice is weak without stridor, there is no dyspnea and no force to coughing, and dysphagia is present.

How to Look at the Vocal Cords

1. Use a round dental mirror, 15–20 mm in diameter, on an 8-in handle. Warm it under hot tap water and dry it.
2. Ask the patient to open his mouth, sit still, and breathe through his mouth. Hold his tongue down with a tongue blade held in your left hand. This hand holds the penlight on top of the tongue blade as shown in Figure 9–2.
3. Put the warm (not hot) mirror far enough back in the pharynx until you can see down the larynx and can see the vocal cords. Ask the patient to say "eh, eh" and "ah, ah" several times.

Compare the amount and speed of movement of the two cords. If touching his palate or pharynx with the mirror makes him gag, a little lidocaine spray will temporarily abolish the afferent side of the gag reflex. If you use a cold mirror, water vapor will condense on it and you will see nothing.

Things to Remember About Cranial Nerves 9 and 10

- Can the patient swallow liquids and solids?
- Is there nasal regurgitation or coughing when he swallows?
- Is the voice different in any way?
- Can the patient cough forcefully?
- An absent gag reflex (bilateral) is often normal; a unilaterally absent gag reflex is not normal.

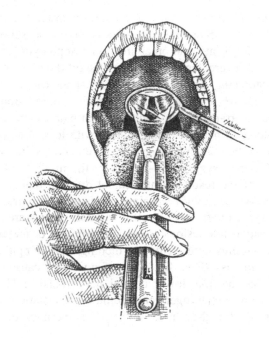

Figure 9–2. To examine the larynx, hold the penlight and tongue blade (taped together) in your left hand and the warm mirror in your right.

- Is the speech "bubbly"? Does the patient have trouble clearing mucus from his cords?

Diseases Affecting Nerves 9 and 10

These diseases may be

- Central—Brain stem infarct, syringobulbia, glioma, poliomyelitis, and amyotrophic lateral sclerosis
- At the base of the brain—Chronic meningitis, meningioma, aneurysm, acoustic neuroma, and Wegener's granulomatosis
- Peripheral—Perforating injury to the neck, enlarged tracheobronchial nodes, aortic aneurysm, and mediastinal mass lesions
- Miscellaneous—Myasthenia gravis may present with progressive weakness of the voice. The more the patient talks, the weaker the voice gets, with or without dysphagia. Oculopharyngeal dystrophy is sometimes more pharyngeal and less ocular in terms of complaints.
- Pseudobulbar palsy—Can present with abnormalities of speech, chewing,

and swallowing, but the lesion is not in the ninth or tenth cranial nerve

- Both the ninth and tenth cranial nerves convey some sensation from the external ear, posterior palate, and other areas. Glossopharyngeal neuralgia consists of attacks of severe, lancinating pain of short duration and is commonly induced by swallowing. The pain is in the throat and ear, has the same qualities as tic douloureux, and may be symptomatic of nerve trunk compression (neuroma or an aberrant vessel). Each attack of pain can be accompanied by a transient change in heart rate and rhythm with loss of consciousness (the carotid branch of the glossopharyngeal nerve innervates the carotid sinus).
- The jugular foramen syndrome—Lesion of the ninth, tenth, and eleventh cranial nerves. If the result of intracranial disease, there is usually brain stem compression and long tract signs. If caused by extracranial disease, the cervical sympathetic and twelfth cranial nerves are frequently involved. The responsible lesions are usually primary or metastatic tumor of the skull base, glomus jugulare tumor, meningioma, or epidermoid tumors.
- Polyneuritis cranialis—This disease is of unknown cause. It starts in elderly patients as multiple lower cranial nerve palsies. They are usually thought to have nasopharyngeal carcinoma or metastatic carcinoma at the base of the skull, but they have neither. It sometimes improves spontaneously.
- Diphtheria and botulism toxins—Both can cause bulbar palsy

ELEVENTH NERVE

The eleventh (spinal accessory) nerve is a motor nerve that originates intracranially in the medulla and also in the cervical spinal cord. It is both a cranial nerve and a spinal nerve. It innervates the sternomastoid muscle and the upper portion of the trapezius muscle.

How to Test the Spinal Accessory Nerve If you have the patient face you, put your hand on the right side of his head as in Figure 9–3A, and ask him to turn to the right against the resistance of your hands, you will *not* learn anything. You cannot see or feel the left sternomastoid effectively.

> However, if you ask him to turn his head to the right as far as he can, unresisted, and then you attempt to bring the head back to the facing position against his resistance, you will see, as in Figure 9–3B, the size of the left sternomastoid and feel the strength of it.

To test the trapezius,

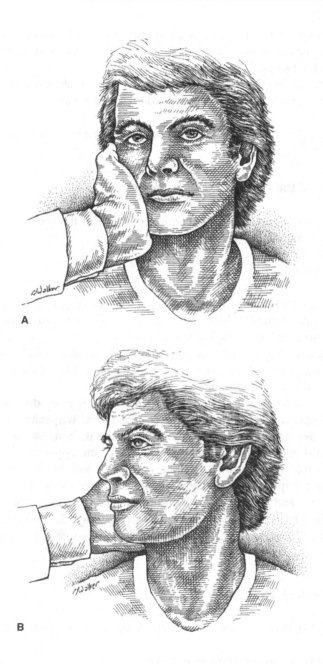

Figure 9–3. A. The *wrong* way to examine the left sternomastoid. The patient attempts to turn his head to his right against resistance. **B.** The *correct* way to examine the left sternomastoid. The patient turns his head to the right unresisted. The examiner then attempts to bring the head back to the forward position as the patient resists.

• Stand behind the patient. Look at the patient's neck, back, and shoulders. Do they appear to be symmetrical, and are the muscles the same size and bulk on the two sides?
• Hold the upper edge of the muscle between your thumb and fingers and ask him to shrug his shoulders upward toward the ears.

Compare the speed, size (thickness), and strength of the right and left sides.

Diseases of the Eleventh Cranial Nerve

• The jugular foramen lesions mentioned above in the section on the ninth and tenth cranial nerves are important.

Others include

• Lesions in the region of the foramen magnum, upper spinal cord, lower end of the medulla, both extrinsic (neurofibroma) and intrinsic (poliomyelitis), and amyotrophic lateral sclerosis
• Muscular dystrophy, especially myotonic dystrophy, which may present with almost no visible sternomastoid muscle. Myasthenia gravis and polymyositis are also important.
• An upper motor neuron lesion in the hemisphere may produce weakness of the **ipsilateral sternomastoid** and **contralateral trapezius**. With a **pontine upper motor neuron** lesion the **contralateral sternomastoid** is weak. Although still somewhat controversial, the upper motor neuron respecting the sternomastoid originates either in both hemispheres or, more likely, in the ipsilateral hemisphere and decussates twice, that is, to the opposite pons and back again to the same side of the cord as the hemisphere of origin. The upper motor neuron fibers respecting the trapezius appear to originate in the contralateral hemisphere and decussate only once.

TWELFTH NERVE

The twelfth (hypoglossal) nerve is the motor nerve to the tongue.

How to Examine the Hypoglossal Nerve

1. **Have the patient open her mouth without protruding the tongue.** Look in her mouth. How thick is the tongue? Is it flat, wrinkled, mov-

ing, or still? A wasted tongue will appear to be *lower* in the mouth than the normal tongue. Is the midline of the tongue in the midline of the mouth?

2. **Have the patient push her tongue straight out of her mouth.** In some diseases the tongue cannot be protruded beyond the teeth. The tongue normally comes out in the midline. If one half of the tongue is weak or paralyzed, the tongue will always come out of the mouth *to the weak side*, irrespective of whether it is an upper or lower motor neuron lesion.

> In milder degrees of weakness it may be necessary to have the patient push her tongue into her cheek while you hold your finger outside the cheek. Do this on both the right and left sides (Figure 9–4).

Most normal people can extend the tongue from the mouth for about one third to one half its length. The tongue can also be alternatively protruded

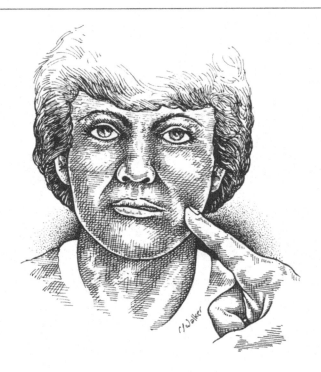

Figure 9–4. To test the strength of the tongue, the patient pushes it into the cheek against the examiner's finger on the right and then on the left.

and withdrawn back into the mouth rapidly. This "trombone" movement of the tongue is normal and becomes slower and abnormal in some diseases.

> Ask the patient to protrude her tongue and then wiggle it from side to side.

When you know how most people do this, you will quickly recognize abnormal tongue movements.

> Ask the patient to rapidly repeat the sound "la-la-la-la."

Parkinsonism, cerebellar lesions, or weakness and wasting of the tongue will make the sound abnormal.

Diseases of the Twelfth Cranial Nerve

Most bilateral lesions of the tongue are the result of amyotrophic lateral sclerosis. (See also the lower cranial nerves described above.)

The Upper Limb

10

The arm is between the shoulder and the elbow; the forearm is between the elbow and the wrist.

Assessment of upper limb function may be **directed** when the patient says, for example, "I have a pain in my right neck and shoulder and numbness in my fingers and I drop things from my right hand." He must have a disease of the spinal cord, canal, root, or brachial plexus. The nature of his complaint thus will direct your thinking.

When there are direct symptoms, try to convert these into defects of function. If the patient says, "My hand is numb," then you will want to ask, "Does bath [dish] water feel equally hot on both your hands? Can you put your hand in your pocket [purse] and bring out a key or a coin and know what it is without first looking at it? Has your handwriting changed? Can you tie your necktie [put your earrings or contact lenses in] as well as you used to? Can you do up buttons, zippers, or hooks and sew, type, play the guitar, and work your personal computer as well as you always could?"

Also, remember that *numbness* implies a sensory disorder when doctors use the word, but not so with patients. Patients with pure motor lesions, basal ganglion disorders, and other nonsensory lesions sometimes describe the affected part as "numb."

In contrast is the **undirected** assessment of upper limb function. The patient's family, or perhaps his employer, says, "He cannot do his office work as well as he could a year ago. He seems to shuffle a bit when he walks, and he does not stand up straight anymore." What has this to do with the arms? While you are taking the patient's history, you notice that his right arm has not lifted off the armrest of the chair once in 30 min. When he emphasizes spoken speech with a gesture, only the left hand "does the talking." All the normal, small, useless movements such as adjusting the knot in the necktie, sliding the glasses up onto the nose, or rubbing the cheek with a finger are done with the left hand. The patient has parkinsonism. The most obvious physical sign is the immobility of the right upper limb. Once you have thought of the diagnosis, you make your inquiries from a different perspective, and yes, the patient, on reflection, admits that his handwriting *is* different in the past 2 years and, yes, the newspaper *does* appear to tremble on occasion when he is tired and holding it up in front of him. But the presenting complaints were a gait disorder and inability to perform on the job; the right upper limb was supposedly symptom-free.

The most important things to look at during history taking in any patient are the face, the stance, and the upper limbs. While the patient answers questions, watch him. Similarly, do not let anyone else go to get your patient from the waiting area. Get him yourself, then watch the patient as you introduce yourself and as he gets out of the chair, goes with you to the consulting room, sits, and gets ready to tell his story.

If he gets out of the chair by pushing down on the chair arms or on his knees with his hands, his quadriceps are weak. If he seems to rock back and forth in the chair two or three times before "launching" himself to stand, he is stiff because of parkinsonism, medication, or some other cause. Do his arms swing as he walks? Does his right arm come forward synchronously with his left leg? Are there excessive, random, restless, small movements of the hands and arms, suggesting chorea? Is there a repetitive, stereotyped hand-and-arm movement such as wiping the lips every 15 s, as one might see in a patient with tardive dyskinesia?

POSTURAL MAINTENANCE

When the examination of cranial nerves and visual fields is complete and the patient is still sitting on the examining table with his legs hanging over the side, do the following:

- Ask him to hold his arms out in front of him at shoulder level (loosely, not rigid) with a few degrees of flexion at the elbow, his fingers separated, and the palms uppermost.
- Then ask him to close his eyes (Figure 10–1) and watch him for 10 or 15 s.

If one arm begins to drift down toward the floor or down and out, or occasionally up, this is evidence of organic disease. The test is not specific but it is *objective*. The disease may be in the sensory system (ipsilateral or contralateral), the contralateral basal ganglia, upper motor neuron system, or ipsilateral cerebellum.

If both arms drift toward the floor, the test is uninformative. The patient does not understand or he is tired, obtunded, on drugs, or ill in a generalized way.

If neither arm drifts, gently tap first one arm and then the other to the side and then toward the floor. As you do this, ask the patient to keep his arms in their original position and not allow you to dislodge them. If one arm is

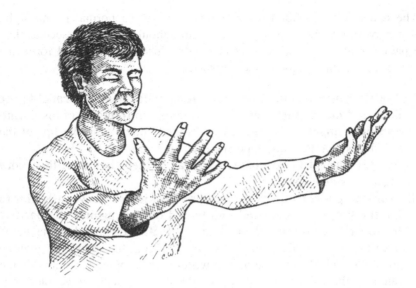

Figure 10–1. To examine the arms for drift, start with them in this position, with the patient's eyes closed.

more easily displaced than the other, this is of the *same* significance as **spontaneous arm drift**.

ALTERNATING MOVEMENTS

The patient's ability to perform alternative movements with the upper limbs can be specifically abnormal, as in cerebellar disease or parkinsonism. Alternating movements may be nonspecifically abnormal in upper motor neuron lesions or with a parietal lobe sensory defect or in the presence of dyskinesia. Testing rapid alternating movements is most informative when they are normal on one side of the body but not on the other.

1. **With the patient sitting and his eyes open, ask him to touch his nose with the tip of his index finger (Figure 10–2A) and then, with the same finger, reach out and touch your finger.** Keep your hand still. Ask the patient to do this two or three times. Carefully watch the last 10–15 cm of movement of the patient's finger as he approaches his nose and your finger. The **terminal intention tremor**, diagnostic of cerebellar disease, is best seen in this portion of the movement.

The patient's hand-and-arm movement may appear normal in midflight, and it may appear more or less normal throughout the first or second time the patient does it. As he persists in moving his hand back and forth, the tremor increases and becomes more obvious.

2. **Ask the patient to hold his arms at shoulder height parallel to the floor and make quick, repetitive, pinching movements of his thumb and little finger.** This should be a "round" pinch with the tips of the two digits, not the pads, opposing each other (Figure 10–2B).
3. **Ask the patient to do this with one arm, then the other, then both together, side by side.**
4. **With the patient's arms in the same position as above, ask him to tap the fingers of one hand lightly and quickly against the back of the other, then reverse them (Figure 10–2C).** You will learn as much from listening to this as from watching it. From the sound you may be able to tell which hand the patient writes with. Tapping is commonly the same in the two hands. If the dominant hand taps slower and less adroitly than the nondominant one, then the dominant limb is abnormal.

Single hand clapping (Figure 10–2D) should also be watched and listened to.

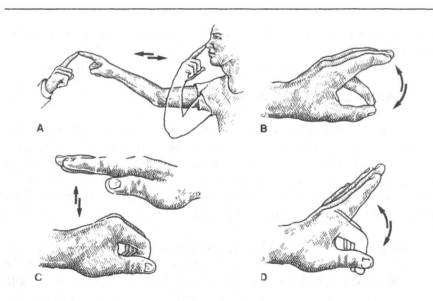

Figure 10–2. Tests of rapid alternating movements. **A.** Finger-nose-finger testing. **B.** Pinching the thumb and the little finger together (the thumb and the index finger can also be used). **C.** Tapping one hand on the back of the other. **D.** One-hand clapping.

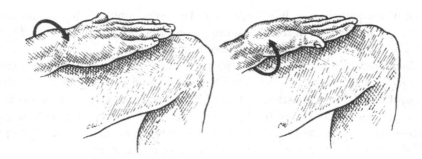

Figure 10–3. A further test of upper limb coordination. Rapid alternating prone-supine-prone positions of the hand on the thigh.

Finally, as shown in Figure 10–3,

5. **Have the patient put his hand, palm up, on his thigh and rotate it, prone-supine-prone, several times.** He should make the dorsal and volar surface contact his thigh each time so that you hear the slap. Ask him to do this with one hand, then the other.

All of these tests should take no more than 35–60 s. In the presence of slight degrees of incoordination, weakness, sensory loss, or basal ganglion disease, the abnormalities of rapid alternating movement may be evident only in the performance of one arm *relative* to the other; that is, the function of the limb is abnormal only by comparison. These tests are of greatest value in establishing **lateralization** and **organicity**.

They do not help much, however, in assessing the patient with the obvious spastic arm. A spastic limb will have abnormal rapid alternating movements and coordination, and the spasticity may be the only explanation. Also, the spasticity may prevent you from eliciting the signs of cerebellar ataxia or tremor. Similarly, these tests are not too helpful in the examination of someone with a dyskinesia or involuntary movements. The involuntary movements interfere with the consecutive repetitive parts of any of the rapid alternating movements.

TONE

Muscle tone is defined as the **resistance to passive stretching**. The tone of the normal, relaxed, resting limb is difficult to identify and distinguish from that of the pathological hypotonic limb. However, after you have examined several patients with flaccid, hypotonic limbs that feel like the arms and legs of a rag doll, you will know the tone of normal limbs.

Increased tone is not difficult to identify. The resistance may be greatest at the start of stretching and then vanish as the muscle is lengthened, as with a clasp knife. This is **spasticity**. In cerebral lesions it is greatest (and earliest in a progressive lesion) in the flexor muscles of the *upper* limb and the extensor muscles of the *lower* limb, but not confined to these muscle groups. When the lesion is spinal, the distribution is more variable.

Rigidity is the term used for increased tone resulting from disease of the basal ganglia. It may be **plastic**, in which the resistance is uniform throughout stretching, that is, like bending a piece of soldering wire, or **cogwheel**. In the latter, as the muscle is stretched the examiner feels resistance, relaxation, resistance, and so on, throughout the stretch. Rigidity is not more evident in one muscle group than in another and, unlike spasticity, is greatest or greater in the trunk than in the limbs.

Increased tone from any cause can often be easily exhausted by several consecutive stretches. If the muscle being examined is then put at rest, the increased tone can be felt again. In the upper limb it is important to assess tone in the fingers and at the wrist, elbow, and shoulder.

1. **Take the patient's hand in your hand with her palm toward the floor, your thumb in the middle of her palm, and your fingers on the dorsum of her hand. With your other hand, gently and quickly extend all of her fingers together at the metacarpal phalangeal joints.**
2. **When the patient's fingers have been extended as far as they can go comfortably, let go of them. They will naturally resume a flexed position. Then stretch them again.** Do this several times. There are no diseases in which increased tone is manifest in the finger extensors more than or earlier than the finger flexors. Therefore, you need not stretch the extensors.
3. **To test at the wrist, hold the forearm in one hand and passively extend the patient's wrist as you did the fingers. After each extension let the hand fall back into a flexed position, and repeat the passive stretching quickly several times. You may elicit wrist clonus by doing this** (see the section on "Clonus" in Chapter 13).

There is another method to get the sense of the tone in the patient's forearm muscles.

4. **Hold the supine patient's forearm vertically, with her elbow flexed to 90 degrees and her fingers toward the ceiling. Let your fingers**

and thumb surround the patient's forearm about halfway between her wrist and elbow. Ask the patient to relax the wrist as much as possible. Then shake her forearm from side to side. In a person with normal tone the hand flops from side to side on the end of the forearm. The first time you try this on a patient with parkinsonism or an upper motor neuron lesion, you will at once recognize an increase in tone.

5. **At the patient's elbow, stretch the flexors starting from a position of extreme elbow flexion. Stretch the flexors by rapidly extending the forearm several times.** Remember, at metacarpophalangeal and interphalangeal joints and at the wrist and elbow, increases in tone are *earliest* and *most evident* in the flexors as opposed to the extensor muscles.

In an early upper motor neuron lesion, an increase in tone in the upper limb may occur first in the **pronator muscles** of the forearm. Test for it this way:

6. **As shown in Figure 10–4, have the patient lie on his back, with his elbow flexed at a right angle and his forearm across his trunk. If you are standing on the right side of the examining table (as shown in the figure), take the patient's left hand in your left hand while his forearm is prone across his chest. Rapidly supinate and pronate his forearm several times while keeping his elbow flexed and his forearm across his trunk.** The stretching of the pronator muscles may elicit pronator clonus, and if there is increased tone, it is unmistakable when examined this way.

SIZE

1. **Measure the circumference of the patient's forearm and arm, right and left, *where the circumference is greatest* and record the measurements in your notes.** Have the arm in full extension. Figure 10–5 shows the positions. Do not pick arbitrary distances distal and proximal to the elbow and then measure the circumference at these points. Many people have a larger forearm and arm on the dominant side, but the difference is usually not more than 5–10 mm.

2. **Look and feel the small muscles of the patient's hands when looking at the *thenar* and *hypothenar eminences*. Always adduct all fingers and the thumb.** This "rounds" the thenar eminence and shows it to its best advantage.

3. **Look at the dorsum of the hand, noting the prominence of the extensor tendons.** These will be more obvious in one hand than the other if there is small muscle wasting in the former.

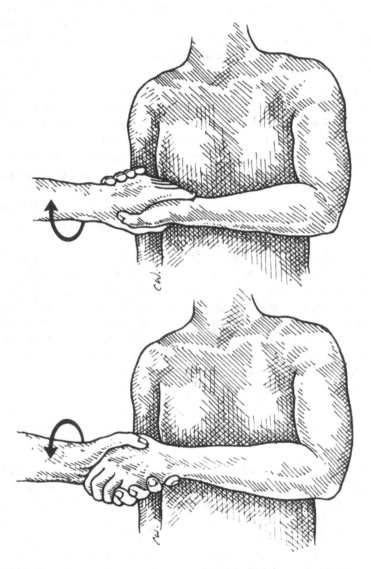

Figure 10–4. To test pronator muscle tone with the patient supine, grasp the patient's hand and quickly pronate and supinate the forearm.

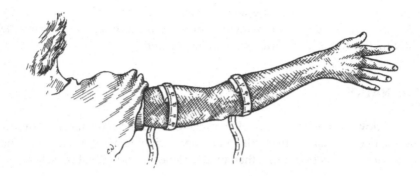

Figure 10–5. Measure the circumferences of the forearm and the arm where they are greatest.

In the normal male hand, if the thumb is *adducted*, the first dorsal interosseous muscle bulges up on the dorsal surface. It may be flat, but it is never a dimple or depression. Feel the muscle as shown in Figure 10–6.

4. *Extend* **the patient's thumb, feel the web of skin between his finger and thumb, and keep moving your examining fingers proximally (as shown in the figure) in small, gentle pinches until you have the full thickness of his first dorsal interosseous between the tips of your thumb and index finger.** You can identify a wasted first dorsal interosseous muscle far earlier by this method than by looking at it.

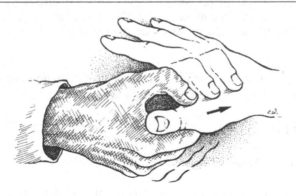

Figure 10–6. Feel the bulk and size of the patient's first dorsal interosseous muscle. While the patient extends his thumb, make a series of gentle pinches with your thumb and index finger in the direction of the arrow.

Upper limb size can be assessed when testing arm drift (Figure 10–1). Look down the length of the patient's arms from the fingertips toward the chest. Small differences in arm size will be apparent.

EXAMINATION

The following are the minimal number of muscles you must examine. With practice you can do them all and compare right and left in minutes. The headings are by function rather than by the names of individual muscles.

Abduction of the Fingers

Dorsal Interossei: Ulnar Nerve, T1

> With the palm of the patient's hand on a flat surface, ask him to spread his fingers against resistance.

The first dorsal interosseous (see step 4 of the previous section and Figure 10–6) is easy to see and feel as the index finger is abducted. The abductor of the little finger is just as distinctive on the ulnar border of the hand.

Abduction of the Thumb

Abductor Pollicis Longus: Radial Nerve, C7; Abductor Pollicis Brevis: Median Nerve, T1

> Put the dorsum of the patient's hand on a flat surface. Ask him to raise the thumb vertically. The surface of the pad of the thumb is at right angles to the surface of the palm of the hand.

The **brevis** is part of the thenar eminence, and the tendon of the **longus** can be seen and felt on the lateral side of the wrist.

Opposition of the Thumb

Opponens Pollicis: Median Nerve T1

> As shown in Figure 10–7, ask the patient to push the pad of his thumb against the pad of his little finger. Try to separate them with your index finger, moving in the direction of the arrow shown in the figure.

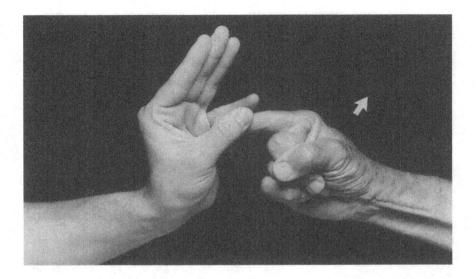

Figure 10–7. Testing the strength of the patient's left opponens pollicis. The thumb and the little finger are opposed (not flexed). The examiner moves his finger in the direction of the arrow.

Do not let the patient *flex* the tip of the thumb against the tip of his little finger.

Flexion of the Fingers

Flexor Digitorum Profundus*: Ulnar and Anterior Interosseous Nerve, a Branch of the Median Nerve, C8

Ask the patient to place the *dorsum* of his hand on a flat surface as shown in Figure 10–8. He should attempt to flex the terminal phalanx of each finger while you fix the middle phalanx as shown in Figure 10–8A.

Flexor Digitorum Sublimis (or Superficialis): Median Nerve (All), C8

Have the patient flex his middle phalanx against resistance while you fix the proximal phalanx, as shown in Figure 10–8B.

---

* The two lateral flexors related to the index and middle fingers are supplied by the **anterior interosseous branch** of the **median nerve**; the other two, by the **ulnar nerve**.

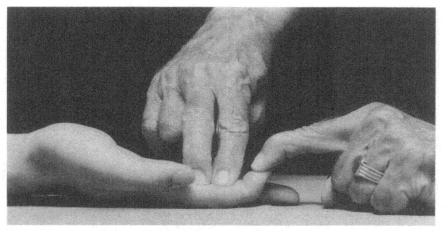

A

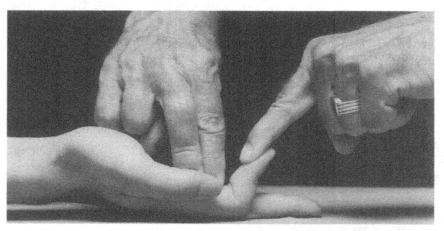

B

Figure 10–8. A. The flexor digitorum profundus is tested for strength as the examiner attempts to extend the distal phalanx of each finger in succession. **B.** The flexor digitorum sublimis is tested as the patient flexes the middle phalanx against resistance.

The profundus flexors can take part in this as well as the sublimis. *Remember:*

        Profundus are **P**eripheral
        Sublimis are **S**hort

Flexion of the Wrist

Flexor Carpi Ulnaris: Ulnar Nerve, C8; Flexor Carpi Radialis: Median Nerve, C8

Ask the patient to put the dorsum of his hand and forearm on a flat surface and flex his wrist against resistance as shown in Figure 10–9.

With wrist flexion plus a little *abduction* the tendon of the flexor carpi radialis in the midline of the wrist is seen (arrow in Figure 10–9A), while with flexion plus a little *adduction* the flexor carpi ulnaris becomes palpable on the most *medial* aspect of the wrist (Figure 10–9B).

The tendon of the flexor carpi ulnaris can also be seen and felt on the medial wrist by *abducting* the little finger.

Flexion of the Forearm

Biceps: Musculocutaneous Nerve, C5 and C6; Brachioradialis: Radial Nerve, C6

To test the biceps, have the patient's forearm and hand on a flat surface with the dorsal aspect of the limb touching the surface. Fix his elbow and ask him to flex his forearm against resistance.

To test the brachioradialis, start from the same position except that the forearm is halfway between supine and prone; that is, the ulnar edge of the hand and forearm is resting on a flat surface and the thumb is uppermost. Ask the patient to flex his forearm against resistance from this position.

These two powerful forearm flexors have the same root supply and different nerve supply.

Flexion of the Thumb

Flexor Pollicis Longus: Anterior Interosseous Nerve, a Branch of the Median Nerve, C8

Hold the proximal phalanx of the patient's thumb between your finger and thumb. This provides a fixed base. Then have the patient flex the *distal* phalanx against resistance.

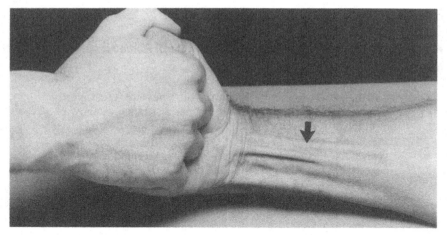

A

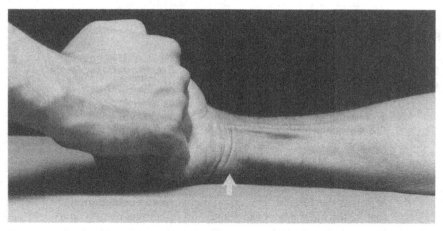

B

Figure 10–9. The forearm is supine and the dorsal surface is supported on the examining table. **A.** To test the flexor carpi *radialis*, the patient flexes and abducts the wrist. The tendon of the muscle is in the midvolar aspect of the wrist at the arrow. **B.** To test the flexor carpi *ulnaris*, the patient flexes and abducts the wrist. The tendon is palpable on the medial aspect of the wrist at the arrow.

Flexor Pollicis Brevis   Supply here is both median and ulnar, although it is most often ulnar only (T1). The ambiguity of innervation makes examination unrewarding.

Extension of the Thumb

Extensor Pollicis Longus and Extensor Pollicis Brevis, Both Supplied by the Posterior Interosseous Nerve, a Branch of the Radial Nerve, C7

Have the patient put the ulnar edge of his hand and forearm on a flat surface, with the hand midway between prone and supine and the thumb extended vertically. If resistance is applied to the distal phalanx, the *longus* is being tested. If resistance is applied to the proximal phalanx, the *brevis* is being tested.

The tendons of these two muscles plus the tendon of the abductor pollicis longus make up the sides of the "snuff-box" on the radial edge of the wrist.

Extension of the Fingers

Extensor Digitorum: Posterior Interosseous Nerve, a Branch of the Radial Nerve, C7

As shown in Figure 10–10, ask the patient to keep his hand and wrist stiff and prone. Use the edge of your left hand as a

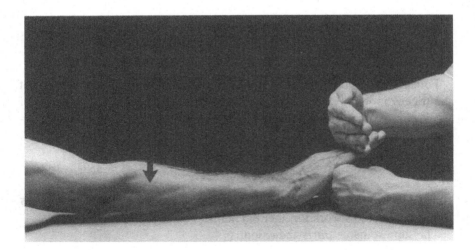

Figure 10–10. The extensor digitorum is tested using the examiner's hand as a fulcrum. The patient rigidly extends his fingers, and the examiner attempts flexion at the metacarpophalangeal joints. The muscle belly is at the arrow.

fulcrum in the middle of the patient's palm. Attempt to flex the patient's fingers with your right hand.

The extensors function at the **metacarpal phalangeal joints.** Extension at the more distal interphalangeal joints is performed by the interossei and lumbricales.

Extension of the Wrist

Extensor Carpi Radialis (Longus and Brevis): Radial Nerve, C7 and C8;
Extensor Carpi Ulnaris: Posterior Interosseous Nerve, a Branch
of the Radial Nerve, C7 and C8

The radialis is tested as in Figure 10–11A. Place the volar aspect of the forearm on any flat surface. Allow some flexion of the fingers at the interphalangeal and metacarpophalangeal joints in order to get the finger extensors relaxed and out of the way. Then ask the patient to forcefully extend and abduct the hand while you supply resistance to the dorsum of the hand. The ulnaris is examined by having the patient extend and adduct his hand (Figure 10–11B).

Extension of the Forearm

Triceps: Radial Nerve, C7

Allow the patient to flex his elbow to form about a 90-degree angle at the elbow and then straighten his arm against resistance.

Forearm extension is never as strong as forearm flexion. If you want to put the triceps in its most disadvantageous position and elicit small amounts of weakness, ask the patient to begin forearm extension from a position of maximum elbow flexion.

Abduction of the Arm

Supraspinatus: Suprascapular Nerve, C5; Deltoid: Axillary Nerve, C5
These two muscles work together but neither can do the job of the other.
The supraspinatus *starts* abduction.

Test the supraspinatus by standing behind the patient. He should let his arms hang by his sides. Hold his elbow into the side of his trunk while he attempts to abduct the arm.

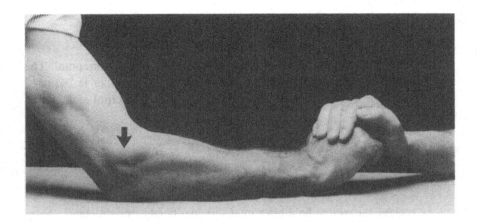

A

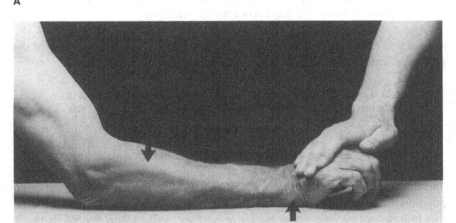

B

Figure 10–11. A. Extension and abduction at the wrist reveals the extensor carpi radialis (arrow). **B.** Extension and adduction reveals the extensor carpi ulnaris. The arrow shows the muscle (left), and the tendon can be felt at the right arrow.

You may feel the muscle above the spine of the scapula. The trapezius lies on top of it and you cannot always see it or feel it.

If either the **trapezius** or **supraspinatus** is wasted, there is a trough or depression above the spine of the scapula.

If the patient cannot *fix* the scapula (see the subsections on the trapezius muscle, rhomboids, and serratus anterior in the section on "Fixation of the Scapula," below), it is difficult to be certain of supraspinatus weakness.

Test the deltoids by resisting abduction after the arm has
been abducted 45 degrees and more away from the trunk.

The deltoid is working most effectively when the arm is horizontal. The
muscle is easily seen and felt. When it is wasted, the shoulder is "square"
when looking at it from in front or behind. This is the **principal** abductor of
the arm.

Adduction of the Arm

Latissimus Dorsi: Thoracodorsal Nerve, C7

Have the patient hold his arm at shoulder height straight out
to one side, parallel to the floor. Ask him to put his hand on
your shoulder and push down toward the floor.

Examine the anterior and posterior axillary walls. The *lower portion* of the
posterior wall of the axilla is the latissimus dorsi.

You may also test it by holding it between your finger and
thumb while the patient has his arms at his side. Then ask
him to cough.

You will feel the edge of the latissimi contract between your fingers.

Teres Major: Subscapular Nerve, C7
Start with the patient's arm in the same
position as above (arm parallel to the floor at shoulder height). You can see
this muscle only in the upper posterior axillary wall in thin people. It is off
the lateral edge of the scapula and posterior to the upper end of the latissimus.

Pectoralis Major: Clavicular Part—Lateral Pectoral Nerve, C5; Sternal Part— Lateral and Medial Pectoral Nerve, C7, C8, and T1

Ask the patient to put one fist against the other and push as
in Figure 10–12.

Fixation of the Scapula
A wing scapula and resulting weak shoulder are common complaints. The
three principal muscles concerned with fixation and movement of the
scapula have overlapping functions.

Trapezius Muscle: Spinal Accessory Nerve, C3 and C4
The trapezius pulls
the scapula *upward*. This was demonstrated in the "shoulder shrug" when

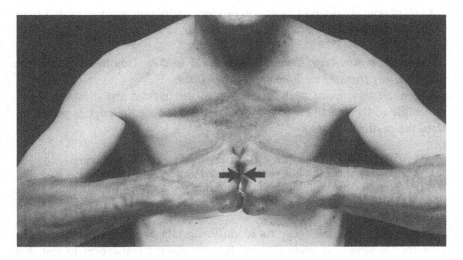

Figure 10–12. Test the pectoralis muscle by asking the patient to push one fist against the other. The muscle has two heads, the clavicular and the sternal.

you examined the eleventh cranial nerve (see "How to Test the Spinal Accessory Nerve" in Chapter 9). It also pulls the medial edge of the scapula toward the midline (**adduction**). Therefore, if only trapezius weakness is the cause of the wing scapula, the scapula is lower and more *lateral* when the shoulder is at rest.

> Ask the patient to abduct his arm away from his trunk against resistance. The *downward* and *lateral* displacement of the scapula will be more obvious and the winging is most obvious at the lower edge.

> Ask the patient to put his arms horizontally straight in front of him as though pushing the wall (flexion); the winging disappears (compare with serratus anterior palsy).

Rhomboids: Dorsal Scapular Nerve, C5 These muscles pull the medial edge of the scapula *upward* and *toward the midline.* You "brace" the shoulders with your rhomboids.

> To see normal rhomboid function, ask the patient to put his hand on his hip and push his elbow backward against the resistance of the examiner's hand. Watch and feel the medial edge of the scapula move *toward the midline and upward.*

In rhomboid weakness this action produces winging, and the medial edge of the scapula moves laterally and downward.

Serratus Anterior: Long Thoracic Nerve, C5 to C7 This muscle pulls the scapula *away from the midline* and also *forward.*

When the serratus is weak, inspection of the back at rest shows the *inferior* angle of the scapula is slightly *winged* and the medial edge is pulled toward the midline.

> Abduction of the arm against resistance *reduces* the winging. Pushing the horizontally flexed arm against the wall *increases* the winging, and the inferior angle of the scapula is lifted off the chest wall.

Remember: The *best* test to identify scapula winging resulting from *trapezius* weakness is *abduction* of the arm against resistance; to test that caused by *serratus anterior* weakness, use *flexion* (with the arm horizontal, pushing forward against the wall).

UPPER LIMB ABNORMALITIES

The upper limb is of about the same importance in neurological assessment as eye movements and vision. Diseases of the upper motor neuron, parietal lobe, cerebellum, and basal ganglia may each produce characteristic changes in the tone, power, posture, or function of the limb and are dealt with elsewhere. Diseases of the spinal cord, nerve roots, brachial plexus, and individual nerves present their own distinctive problems. Herewith are a few comments on plexus and peripheral nerve lesions.

Brachial Plexus

Brachial plexus most commonly involves lesions caused by trauma (traction injury to the arm, knife or ice pick wounds, or bullet penetration), metastatic carcinoma from the breast or lung, or delayed radiation damage to the plexus from treatment of the latter. Other causes are birth injuries, supraclavicular pressure during anesthesia, intravenous drug abuse, serum and vaccination reactions, and paralytic brachial neuritis of unknown cause (possibly virus).

1. **Upper trunk lesions** (eg, Duchenne-Erb syndrome); usually a result of perforating injuries
   - Think of functions of the C5–C6 roots.
   - There is weakness of the supraspinatus, infraspinatus, deltoid, biceps, brachialis, brachioradialis, supinator, and extensor carpi longus and brevis.

- The *lateral* aspect of the arm is numb.
- Biceps and supinator reflexes are absent.
- The rhomboids and serratus anterior are usually normal (as their nerves—dorsal scapular and long thoracic, respectively—arise proximal to the common site of injury).

2. **Lower trunk lesions** (eg, Klumpke syndrome); common causes are cervical rib, carcinoma of the lung apex, and metastatic carcinoma in the axillary lymph nodes, as well as traction on the abducted arm
   - Think of functions of the C8 and T1 roots.
   - There is weakness of the flexor carpi ulnaris, flexor digitorum, interossei, and thenar and hypothenar muscles; the hand is flat and simian.
   - The ulnar edge of the arm, forearm, and hand is numb.
   - The triceps reflex is absent.
   - Horner's syndrome is commonly present.

3. **Lateral cord lesions**
   - Think of functions of the musculocutaneous nerve and the *lateral* part of the median nerve.
   - There is weakness of the biceps, brachialis, coracobrachialis, and pronator teres.
   - Intrinsic hand muscles are normal (the *medial* part of the median nerve).
   - The radial edge of the forearm may be numb.
   - The biceps reflex is absent.

4. **Medial cord lesions**
   - Think of functions of the ulnar nerve and the medial part of the median nerve.
   - There is weakness of the flexor carpi ulnaris, all flexor digitorum profundus, all interossei, all lumbricales, and all thenar and hypothenar muscles.
   - There is numbness, usually in the ulnar distribution.

5. **Posterior cord lesions**
   - Think of functions of the radial and axillary nerves.
   - There is weakness of the deltoid, teres minor, brachioradialis and supinator, triceps, extensor carpi (all three), extensor digitorum muscles, and long abductor pollicis.
   - There is numbness in the upper outer aspect of the arm just below the deltoid muscle.

6. **Radial nerve lesions**; the nerve is derived from C6 to C8 (mostly C7)
   - These are caused by the pressure of a crutch, a gunshot, stab wounds, fracture of the humerus, and on the medial aspect of the lower arm from pressure during sleep while intoxicated or sedated ("Saturday night palsy").

- A lesion in the axilla causes weakness of the triceps, brachioradialis, the three extensor carpi, and finger extensors; the triceps reflex is absent.
- The area of numbness (if any) is about a 3-cm circular area overlying the first dorsal interosseous muscle; patients rarely have sensory symptoms.
- The apparent weakness of finger flexion in the "wrist-dropped" hand is not real; if the wrist is passively extended, the flexors are found to be normal.
- Lesions at the midhumerus usually result in a normal triceps muscle.
- Lesions of the posterior interosseous nerve (the final branch of the radial nerve) produce weakness of the extensors of the wrist, index finger, and thumb and are usually caused by entrapment of the nerve where it perforates the supinator muscle.
7. **Median nerve lesions**; the nerve is derived from C5 to T1 (mostly C6)
- These lesions are caused by a dislocated shoulder, stab or gunshot wounds to the proximal nerve, and, more commonly, distal compression in the carpal tunnel at the wrist as part of gout, amyloidosis, acromegaly, arthritis, or an occupational hazard.
- Lesions in the arm cause loss of pronation of the forearm, wrist flexion to the radial side, paralysis of flexion of the thumb and index finger, weakness of flexion of all the other fingers (flexor digitorum sublimis), and paralysis of opposition of the thumb with sensory disturbance over the lateral two thirds of the volar surface of the hand.

Lesions at the wrist cause thenar wasting and weakness with the characteristic sensory loss. The common early complaint is a painful, numb hand that disturbs sleep. Symptoms are relieved by shaking the hand. Pain and numbness are often said to be in *all* fingers and pain is often proximal to the wrist well up into the forearm and arm. While this cannot be explained anatomically, it is heard so often from so many well-motivated patients that it cannot be denied. Patients *always* have sensory symptoms.

8. **Ulnar nerve lesions**; the nerve is derived from C8 and T1
- These are caused by perforating wounds, fractures of the lower end of the humerus, and fractures and dislocation of the olecranon or head of the radius. Symptoms may occur long after an elbow injury. Apparently, minor pressure on the nerve at the elbow as an occupational hazard or in patients confined to full bed rest will produce an ulnar palsy.
- Repeated trauma to the heel of the hand on the ulnar side will traumatize the nerve. The nerve divides into superficial and deep branches in the hand, and the signs of a lesion here are usually entirely motor.

- Lesions at the elbow usually do *not* affect the flexor carpi ulnaris or flexor digitorum profundus 3 and 4, but there is weakness of the abductors and adductors of the fingers, the adductor of the thumb, and lumbricales 3 and 4, and the interossei (particularly the first dorsal) and hypothenar muscles are wasted.
- A complete lesion reveals: half a claw hand with small muscle wasting, the fifth finger held away from the fourth finger, hyperextension at the metacarpophalangeal joints, and flexion at the interphalangeal joints, most marked (the flexion) in the fourth and fifth fingers.
- Sensory disturbance is on the ulnar edge of all of the fifth finger, the ulnar edge or tip of the fourth finger, and the ulnar edge of the palm. Sensory symptoms are never proximal to the wrist (see below for differentiation of a T1 lesion from an ulnar nerve lesion). Patients with ulnar nerve lesions at the elbow *always* have sensory symptoms.

Froment's sign of ulnar palsy can also be a useful indicator. When the patient holds a piece of paper between her thumb and index finger (ie, pinches the piece of paper and pulls), in ulnar palsy the terminal phalanx of the thumb will flex. The adductor pollicis is paretic, and the flexor pollicis longus (median nerve) is functioning in its place.

How to tell the difference between

1. A **C5 root lesion** and an **axillary nerve lesion**: A C5 lesion abolishes *all* abduction of the arm (deltoid and supraspinatus) and causes some weakness of the clavicular head of the pectoralis major, biceps, and brachioradialis muscles. An axillary nerve lesion abolishes only the later part of abduction of the arm (deltoid).
2. A **C6 root lesion** and a **musculocutaneous** or **radial nerve lesion**:
   - A C6 root lesion will cause weakness of the biceps, brachialis, and brachioradialis (*no forearm flexion*) and the extensor carpi radialis.
   - A musculocutaneous root lesion will weaken the biceps and brachialis only. Forearm flexion is carried out by the brachioradialis when the forearm is half supinated. The extensor carpi radialis is normal.
   - A radial nerve lesion will weaken the brachioradialis and extensor carpi radialis. The biceps and brachialis will flex the supine forearm.
3. A **C7 root lesion** and a **radial nerve lesion**:
   - A C7 root lesion will cause weakness of arm adduction (latissimus dorsi), forearm extension (triceps), hand extension (extensor carpi ulnaris), finger extension (extensor digitorum), thumb abduction and extension (abductor pollicis longus and extensor pollicis longus and brevis), and hand flexion (flexor carpi radialis).
   - A radial nerve lesion will produce all of the above *except* that there will be no weakness of the latissimus (thoracodorsal nerve) or of the

flexor carpi radialis (median nerve). In addition, the brachioradialis *will* be paretic.

4. A **T1 root lesion** and an **ulnar nerve lesion**:
   - A T1 root lesion will cause weakness and wasting of *all* the small muscles of the hand.
   - An ulnar nerve lesion will produce a wasted hand, but the $4^{1}/_{2}$ muscles supplied by the first thoracic root and the *median nerve* will be preserved. These are the abductor pollicis brevis, opponens pollicis, first and second lumbricales, and half the flexor pollicis brevis (which may be supplied entirely by the ulnar nerve).

The Lower Limb   **11**

The best screening test of lower limb function is watching the patient walk. Gait and its disorders are discussed in detail in Chapter 12. Go to the waiting area yourself to get your patient, and watch him get out of the chair and walk with you to the examining room. Then watch him sit down.

The leg is between the knee and the ankle; the thigh is between the hip and the knee. The detailed examination of the lower limb is subdivided under the headings of coordination, size, tone, and power.

COORDINATION

All of the tests of coordination are better **lateralizers**, but are less helpful when the legs are equally abnormal.

When the patient is not sure whether one or both legs are abnormal and his history is rather vague—for example, "I cannot walk as well as before" or "I seem to stumble and fall down a lot"—the results of the following tests will be abnormal if the problem is weakness, spasticity, sensory loss, or a cerebellar disorder.

Supine Leg Raising

With the patient supine on the examining table, ask her to lift her leg, with the knee extended, off the table (thigh flexion) as high as she can and then slowly put it down. Have her do this several times with one leg. Then ask her to repeat the movement with the other leg.

If one leg is weak or spastic or has an involuntary movement or a proprioceptive sensory defect, this simple leg-raising test will help you identify it. It is a useful **lateralizer**, if not a **localizer**, and is similar to, but less sensitive than, **arm drift**.

Rapid Alternating Movements

1. With the patient supine, ask him to tap the heel of one foot on the middle of the tibia of the opposite leg, as in Figure 11–1A. The tapping foot should rise 30 cm each time. Watch the rhythm, rate, and regularity

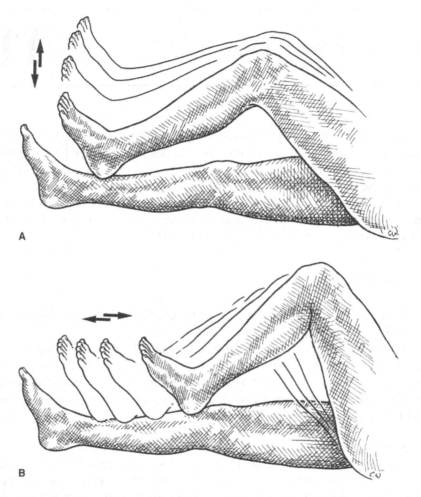

Figure 11–1. Lower limb coordination. **A.** Heel tapping. **B.** Heel sliding.

of this movement and compare the right foot tapping the left tibia and vice versa.

2. Ask the patient to quickly slide the heel of one foot up and down the shin, from knee to ankle, of the opposite leg several times (Figure 11–1B).

Are the rate and rhythm the same, right and left? Or does the right heel, for example, stay on the left tibia throughout the movement while the left heel repeatedly falls off the right tibia?

3. Stand at the foot of the examining table. Put the palm of your hand flat against the sole of the patient's foot, and ask him to tap your hand (ie, move your hand away about 2–3 cm) with his foot repetitively and as quickly as he can. You can do the same thing with the patient sitting by asking him to tap the floor with his foot.

SIZE

Look at the patient's bare legs while he is standing and you are squatting about 2 m from him. Look at him front and back while he stands flat-footed, on his toes, on his heels, and with his kneecaps drawn up (ie, standing at attention).

When you are looking at the back of his legs and he goes up on his toes, a minor amount of calf muscle wasting in one leg will become obvious.

Then, on the examining table, again in the supine position, measure the circumference of the thigh and calf of each leg and write the measurements in the notes.

Measure the leg at its *greatest* circumference, which is at about the junction of the upper and middle thirds. Do *not* measure the circumference at an arbitrary distance below the lower edge of the patella. The greatest circumference of the thigh is usually at the top of the thigh. If you *always* measure the leg and thigh at their *greatest* circumference, there will be no confusion on follow-up examination 6 months or 1 year later.

TONE

Reread the remarks on tone in Chapter 10 on the upper limb and in Chapter 16 on the corticospinal system. When the tone in the legs is increased, watching the patient walk is most revealing.

The bed-bound patient and the patient with *slightly* increased or decreased tone is more difficult to assess.

At times, older patients have an involuntary, normal inability to let the legs relax. Their legs are stiff. They have normal tendon reflexes, plantar responses are down, there is no clonus, and they do not walk with a spastic gait. You may implore such a patient to "just relax" without any change in this resistance of his lower limbs. This phenomenon, called gegenhalten, precludes assessment of lower limb tone.

Assess the tone of the lower limbs as follows:

1. **With the patient supine and his legs straight on the examining table, put your hand in his popliteal fossa. Quickly lift your hand**

toward the ceiling, that is, passively flex the knee. If the quadriceps has normal tone, the heel will usually stay on the examining table as the knee goes up. If the quadriceps is spastic, the heel will lift off the table.

2. **With the patient supine on the table, flex the right hip to a right angle. Hold the thigh in this position with your left hand. Flex the knee to a right angle. The leg is now parallel to the table. Hold the patient's heel in your right hand. Wait a few seconds until he relaxes, then drop the foot while you continue to support the thigh.** If the quadriceps tone is normal, the foot will drop and usually stop just before it hits the table. If the patient is fully relaxed, it will hit the table. If the tone is increased, the foot will drop in a jerky, cogwheel way and never reach the table.

3. **Flex the hip and knee each to about 45 degrees. Externally rotate the hip so that the lateral aspect of the lower limb is resting on the examining table. Rapidly dorsiflex the foot. If the tone is increased in the posterior calf muscles, you will feel the resistance and you may invoke clonus** (see Chapter 13).

POWER

The examination of lower limb power is described with the patient supine and then prone on the examining table. There is also a quick assessment of leg strength with the patient on her feet.

The lower limb muscles are so powerful that *minor* weakness will not be detectable unless you put the muscle in its most disadvantageous position. For example, when you test the tibialis anterior with the patient supine on the table, ask her to actively bend her foot at the ankle and keep her toes up toward her chin while you try to forcefully plantar flex the foot. All you do is slide her down the examining table—you cannot overcome her dorsiflexion. Now have the patient stand up, hold onto a chairback if she needs support, and **stand on her heels**, first with one leg, then the other. The toes of the foot that she is complaining about come off the floor (if at all) by 2 cm. The toes of the normal foot clear the floor by 6 cm.

You now have objective evidence of weakness of dorsiflexion at that ankle. You could not have found this with only the examination on the table.

The order of muscle testing is not anatomical. Start with the iliopsoas and then examine the muscles, from above downward, with the patient supine and then with the patient prone, examined from below upward.

EXAMINATION

Flexion of the Thigh

Iliopsoas Muscle: Spinal Nerves and Femoral Nerve, L2 and L3

With the patient supine, ask him to flex the thigh to a right angle, and then attempt to extend it as he resists, as in Figure 11–2.

Extension of the Leg

Quadriceps Femoris Muscle: Femoral Nerve, L3 and L4

With the thigh flexed at the hip to a right angle and the leg also flexed at the knee to a right angle (or greater than a right angle to elicit minimal quadriceps weakness), ask the patient to straighten his knee against resistance, as in Figure 11–3.

Adduction of the Thigh

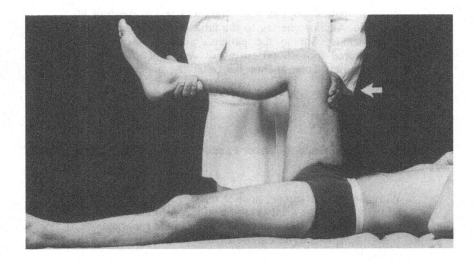

Figure 11–2. Testing the power of the iliopsoas by flexing the hip and knee while the examiner applies force in the direction of the arrow.

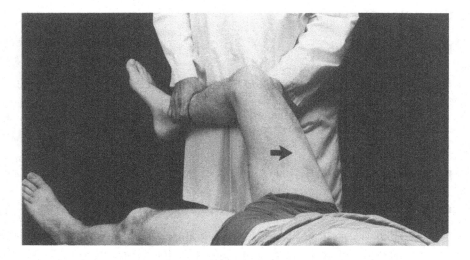

Figure 11–3. Testing the strength of the quadriceps. The patient extends his knee against the examiner's hand. The muscle can be seen to contract (arrow).

Adductor Muscles (Magnus, Longus, and Brevis): Obturator Nerve, L2 and L3

With the patient supine, legs straight, stand at the foot of the table. Anchor one leg to the table by holding it firmly at the ankle. Spread the patient's legs by moving the nonanchored foot 40–60 cm away. Ask him to bring his legs together. Then anchor the other leg and reverse the procedure.

Abduction of the Thigh

Gluteus Medius, Minimus, and Tensor Fascia Lata Muscles: Superior Gluteal Nerve, L4 and L5

With the patient supine, anchor one leg to the examining table by holding it firmly at the ankle. Ask him to move the other leg (the one being tested) away from the anchored one, against resistance. These muscles also act as *medial* rotators of the thigh.

Dorsiflexion of the Foot and Toes

Foot—Tibialis Anterior Muscle: Deep Peroneal Nerve, L4; Big Toe—Extensor Hallucis Longus: Deep Peroneal Nerve, L5; Other Toes—Extensor Digitorum Longus, Deep Peroneal Nerve, L5

> With the patient supine, ask him to vigorously bend his foot toward his head, as in Figure 11–4 (see the section on "Tests" in Chapter 12).

The tendons of these muscles are quite obvious on the dorsum of the foot. The tibialis anterior is a powerful **inverter** of the foot (when the foot is dorsiflexed) as well as a **dorsiflexor**. Therefore, when applying force to overcome it, direct the force toward **plantar flexion and eversion**.

Eversion of the Foot

Peroneus Longus and Brevis Muscles: Superficial Peroneal Nerve, L5 and S1

> With the patient supine and his foot dorsiflexed, ask him to evert the foot as though he were trying to walk on the *inside* edge of his foot. You resist him.

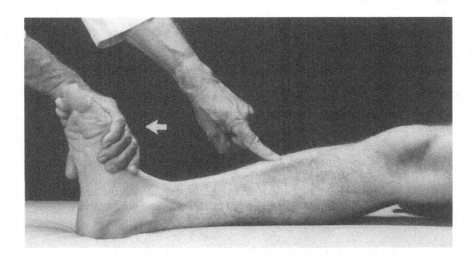

Figure 11–4. Testing the strength of toe and foot dorsiflexion with the patient supine. The examiner plantar flexes against resistance (arrow). The normal tibialis anterior is best seen at its proximal end (at the examiner's finger).

The tendons of the two muscles are seen inferior to the lateral malleolus. These muscles also function as plantar **flexors**.

Inversion of the Foot

Tibialis Posterior Muscle: Tibial Nerve, L4 and L5

With the patient supine and his foot dorsiflexed, ask him to invert his foot as though walking on the *outside* edge of his foot. You resist this movement.

This muscle also acts as a plantar **flexor**.

Plantar Flexion of the Toes

Flexor Digitorum Longus and Flexor Hallucis Longus Muscles: Posterior Tibial Nerve, S1 and S2

Ask the patient to curl his toes downward (plantar flexion) while you resist the movement by pushing upward on the terminal phalanges.

The patient now turns over, and the rest of the examination is conducted in the prone position.

Plantar Flexion of the Foot

Gastrocnemius and Soleus Muscles: Tibial Nerve, S1 and S2

Gastrocnemius—With the patient prone and the knee *extended*, have him attempt to plantar flex his foot against resistance.

This muscle also functions as a flexor of the knee.

Soleus—Have the patient do as above, except that the knee must be *flexed*. Watch and feel the calf muscles while resisting plantar flexion.

Small amounts of weakness of these two muscles may be evident only if the patient is asked to stand on tiptoes, one foot at a time.

Remember, the peroneus (both), the tibialis posterior, and the plantar flexors of the toes assist plantar flexion of the foot.

As you develop your routine of neurological examination, you may find that immediately after testing the soleus is the best time to elicit the ankle reflexes (see Chapter 13).

Leg Flexion at the Knee

Hamstring Muscles (Biceps, Semitendinous, and Semimembranous): Sciatic Nerve, L5 and S1

> With the patient prone, with the knee at a right angle, resist further flexion as the patient attempts to move his heel toward his buttock.

The tendons form the boundaries of the popliteal fossa, the biceps laterally and the semitendinous medially. These muscles also act as **extensors** of the thigh at the hip.

Thigh Extension at the Hip

Gluteus Maximus Muscle: Inferior Gluteal Nerve, L5 and S1

> With the patient prone and the knee extended, ask him to lift the straight leg off the examining table while you press down on the lower posterior thigh (with a weak gluteus maximus the patient will manage to get the leg extended by rotating the pelvis). Make sure he keeps his pelvis on the examining table. You can see and feel the buttock tighten.

This muscle also acts as a **lateral rotator** of the thigh.

Assessment of Leg Strength When the Patient Is on His Feet

- Can he bring the leg forward as he walks?—*iliopsoas*
- Can he get out of a full knee bend without pulling himself up with his arm?—*quadriceps*
- Can he get out of a chair without help from his arm?—*quadriceps* (Parkinsonian rigidity can mimic this.)
- Can he walk on his toes?—*gastrocnemius* and *soleus*
- Can he walk on his heels?—*anterior tibial*
- Does he abduct the leg from the hip and swing it outward and forward to bring the limb ahead instead of the normal thigh flexion (ie, knee drop)?—*all thigh flexors*

- Does he lift one foot much higher from the floor than the other with each step (ie, a foot drop)?—*anterior tibial* and other muscles that are secondarily dorsiflexors

SIGNS AND SYMPTOMS OF SINGLE ROOT LESION

- Second lumbar—Hip flexion weakness is usually the only defect on examination. Pain is in the upper anterior thigh.
- Third lumbar—Hip flexion, knee extension, and thigh adduction are all weak. Pain is in the upper anterior thigh.
- Fourth lumbar—Symptoms of weakness of foot inversion (anterior and posterior tibial muscles) and absent knee reflex. Pain and sensory loss are evident on the medial leg above the malleolus.
- Fifth lumbar—There is weakness of dorsiflexion of the toes, particularly the big toe. Sensory disturbance occurs on the dorsum of the foot; pain is also here and on lateral calf.
- First sacral—Symptoms include weakness of eversion of the foot (peroneii) although innervation is not exclusively first sacral, weakness of plantar flexion of the foot (gastrocnemius and soleus), weakness of leg flexion (hamstring), absent ankle reflex, numbness on the lateral edge of the foot, and pain here and on the back of the calf.

SIGNS AND SYMPTOMS OF NERVE LESIONS

- Lateral cutaneous nerve of the thigh (from L2 and L3)—Painful paresthesias—burning, tingling discomfort in the anterolateral aspect of the thigh—is the only symptom of a disease of this nerve, called meralgia paresthetica. Symptoms are caused by entrapment or stretching of the nerve under the lateral aspect of the inguinal ligament. The disease is common in people who are gaining or losing weight, during or after pregnancy. Symptoms are often related to *one* posture only, such as sitting or standing. Examination reveals hyperesthesia or, rarely, hypoesthesia in the anterior lateral thigh. The thigh is strong, the knee reflex is normal, and disease is benign.
- Obturator nerve (from L2, L3, and L4)—Lesions produce weakness of adduction of the thigh and pain on the medial aspect of the thigh to the knee. The nerve may be injured during delivery or labor or may be involved in pelvic neoplasm.
- Femoral nerve (from L2, L3, and L4)—Lesions produce a wasted quadriceps, weakness of leg extension, and, if the lesion is proximal, weakness of

thigh flexion (iliopsoas muscle) as well. The knee reflex is absent, and sensory loss extends from the anteromedial thigh to the medial malleolus. Diabetes is the most common cause of femoral neuropathy, although pelvic tumors, femoral hernia, and femoral artery aneurysms are also possible causes. A retroperitoneal hematoma may compress the nerve, and drainage of the hematoma is an emergency if the nerve is to be saved.

• Sciatic nerve (from L4 and L5 and S1 and S2)—The lesion will cause loss of knee flexion (hamstrings) and no movement of any muscle below the knee. Sensory loss will occur in all of the **sole of the foot**, the **dorsum of the foot**, and the posterior and lateral leg. Causes are pelvic fractures; penetrating injuries, including misplaced injections; and pelvic tumors. Lying flat on a hard floor while in coma from any cause can produce a compression sciatic palsy.

• Peroneal nerve (the most common peripheral nerve lesion in the lower limb that you will see)—The sciatic nerve divides into the tibial nerve and the common peroneal nerve. The latter winds around the neck of the fibula, a common site of lesions of this nerve. Diabetes, sitting with the legs crossed for long periods, trauma, and sporting injuries (eg, in professional figure skaters or skiers) as well as tightly applied plaster casts account for most of the identifiable causes. There is weakness of dorsiflexion of the toes and foot as well as eversion. The ankle reflex is normal, and although the patient may say he has numbness over the dorsum of the foot, there are usually no sensory abnormalities.

• Posterior tibial nerve (lesions are uncommon)—The nerve may be compromised in its tunnel on the inferomedial aspect of the calcaneus. Pain and paresthesias over the sole of the foot in response to exercise are the only complaints. There are no motor findings.

Stance, Gait, and Balance   12

Walking is an example of the superb integrative action of the nervous system. It is not a learned series of consecutive motor acts but appears as an innate, gestalt phenomenon when other motor skills are still quite primitive, for example, a child may learn to walk at an age when he cannot yet feed himself.

If walking has an anatomical "center," the location is unknown. (Both the cat and the dog can walk after bilateral hemispherectomy.) Walking can be lost, and this may not be explained in terms of a discrete lesion. This is called gait apraxia and is often associated with dementia and frontal lobe signs. However, many demented people have normal gait, and gait apraxia occurs with normal intelligence.

Watch people without gait disorders walk from the front, back, and side.

Considering that the entire weight of the moving body can be continuously transferred from one foot to the other, every three quarters of a second, in a perfectly rhythmic way, without conscious effort, and even while we are preoccupied with some other matter, then walking must be one of the great functions of the nervous system.

When one steps out with the right foot first, three things happen almost simultaneously to the right lower limb. The right hip flexes (the knee comes away from the floor), the right knee flexes (the foot comes away from the floor), and the right ankle plantar flexes in every step except the first one. All the weight is on the left lower limb and, as the right leg comes forward and passes the left, there is more right hip flexion and the beginning of right knee extension and right ankle dorsiflexion in preparation for the transfer of weight to the right heel and foot. While this swing-through of the right leg is progressing, and starting just after the right leg passes the left one, the left ankle plantar flexes in preparation for the push it is about to give to the floor. **Pay particular attention to the foot and ankle movements.** The right heel strikes the floor with the ankle dorsiflexed and the weight of the body on the left foot. As the body comes forward, the right foot flexes and the right lower limb, with the knee extended, takes the weight of the body. The left foot plantar flexes and pushes off against the floor.

The arms reciprocate with the legs. As the left foot comes forward, so does the right upper limb.

> Ask the patient to get out of the chair, walk away from you
> (6–7 m or so), turn quickly to his *left*, and without a pause
> walk back toward you. When he reaches you, have him turn
> quickly to his *right* and repeat the process.

The quick turn may evoke an ataxia not seen otherwise.

TESTS

If ordinary walking is normal, add a number of tests that may elicit an abnormality.

> Have the patient walk a straight line, heel to toe. He should
> put the right heel immediately in front of the left toes and
> then the left heel immediately in front of the right toes and
> so on.

Most people can walk this way across the examining room. If the patient cannot, this itself is not a localizing sign, but it does tell you that something is wrong.

• Have the patient walk on his tiptoes forward across the examining room.
• Ask him to walk on his heels backward across the examining room.
• Ask him to hop across the room on one foot and then the other.

Romberg Test

The Romberg test is named for Moritz Heinrich Romberg (1795–1873). Tradition and your examiners demand that you be familiar with the Romberg test. However, it is *not* a useful or specific way of evaluating ataxia or deciding whether an ataxia is peripheral (sensory) or central (eg, cerebellum).

The basis of the test is the fact that a person with a defect in balance often replaces the *function* of the diseased structure by use of his eyes. If the patient has an ataxic gait because of posterior column disease, peripheral neuritis, or defective sensation for any reason, he may maintain a reasonably good gait provided that he can see the horizon, the walls of the room, or some landmark. The ataxia is more obvious if he closes his eyes or if he is compelled to walk in the dark. The Romberg test is conducted in the following manner:

> The patient is asked to stand with his feet as close together
> as possible while feeling comfortable and stable. He is then
> asked to close his eyes. If he loses his balance, the Romberg
> test is said to be positive.

The tottering *back and forth* that goes on when a person closes his eyes is *not* a positive Romberg. These small, normal movements occur because the patient feels himself leaning toward one side and in correcting it, often over-corrects it, then leans back a little too far the other way, and so forth. When you see this happening, the patient is obviously very much aware of his position in space and has excellent balance. Often, if you say to the patient "Stand perfectly still," the swaying will stop. The patient with a true positive Romberg, on the other hand, is not aware of the beginning of a deviation of his posture and falls over. He makes no attempt to correct it. If he keeps his eyes open, he can maintain a posture; if he closes his eyes, he cannot.

The positive Romberg has been said to be indicative of a **sensory**, or affer-ent, type of ataxia as opposed to a **central**, or cerebellar, type of ataxia. *The conclusion is not valid.* Patients with all kinds of ataxia and with lesions in many different parts of the nervous system will state that they walk reason-ably well indoors, close to walls, in familiar situations. They are much worse out on the street and cannot walk at all in the dark. Therefore, we cannot use the Romberg test to suggest that any given ataxic patient has a sensory lesion as opposed to a central cerebellar lesion.

When a patient complains of being unsteady or stumbling, for example, and on limited examination no evidence of ataxia is found, you may elicit some ataxia by having him stand with his feet together and his eyes shut. In this way the test helps to elicit the physical signs that accompany his symp-toms, but in no sense will it tell you *where* the lesion is.

COMMON DISEASES WITH ABNORMAL GAIT

Parkinsonism

In patients with parkinsonism, walking is slower than normal, cautious, and contained. The steps get smaller and the patient will eventually shuffle. In more advanced disease, she is flexed at the knees and hips and walks on her toes while sliding her feet forward. Her arms are adducted and flexed at the elbow, with her hands held in front of her thigh or abdomen.

Small unevenness of the floor or ground can trip her; her recovery of bal-ance is poor and slow, with frequent falls.

A disturbance of walking or agility of the legs may be the first and *only* complaint in this disease at a time when the patient has no tremor, no visible akinesia, no rigidity, and nothing abnormal about her face or voice.

Cerebellar Disease

Patients with cerebellar disease are ataxic and usually have their feet wide apart. Their gait is irregular in that there will be a short step followed by a long step, a lurch to the right, a long step, a short step, and so on. They often are helped by holding onto another person or a piece of furniture. Perhaps no other gait disorder is improved as much by having an attendant for the patient for the patient to hold as he walks. A *bilateral* cerebellar lesion produces a gait disorder resembling the walk of a drunken person.

Disease of the cerebellar vermis can produce an abnormal gait and balance while limb coordination may be normal.

Unilateral cerebellar hemisphere lesions produce ataxia of gait in the ipsilateral limbs and incoordination toward the side of the lesion. The placement of the ipsilateral foot and lower limb has all the random irregularities seen in both legs in the patient with bilateral disease. The patient may complain that he bumps into people when they walk with him on one side but not on the other. The arm on the side of the cerebellar lesion does not swing. The more acute, large, and recent the lesion, the greater will be the gait disturbance. The cerebellum has great capacity to compensate when it is affected by lesions of slow onset and gradual progression.

Sensory System Disease

Patients with defective proprioception in the legs have an abnormal gait. The lesion may be in the peripheral nerve, posterior root, posterior column, medial lemniscus, or higher.

They also walk with the feet wide apart, watching the floor and landmarks, but are less reeling, lurching, and wild than the patient with cerebellar ataxia. They lift the foot unnecessarily high from the floor and often fling the foot down again, sometimes stopping it before it reaches the floor and other times slapping the floor too forcefully.

These patients are also much worse when walking out of doors, in the dark, or if deprived of vision.

Upper Motor Neuron Disease

Unilateral The hemiplegic gait is identified by arm and leg posture and performance. The arm does not swing and the fingers, wrist, and elbow are flexed. The arm is usually adducted, with the forearm across the abdomen.

The thigh is abducted at the hip, swung out and forward, with fixed plantar flexion and inversion of the foot. There is weakness of both foot dorsiflexion at the ankle and thigh flexion at the hip. For both of these reasons, the entire lower limb is swung out from the hip and then brought forward, thus keeping the toe from dragging on the floor.

Bilateral In bilateral upper motor neuron disease the legs are stiff and the steps are small with the knees adducted and little movement at the ankle, irrespective of which foot is holding the weight or is coming forward. Walking requires a lot of effort, and the toes are often dragged on the floor. There is often a compensating movement of the trunk or upper limbs with each labored movement of the lower limbs.

The apt expression *jiggling* describes a mixed spasticity and cerebellar ataxia and is most frequently seen in patients with multiple sclerosis. The intention tremor of the lower limbs as each foot comes down to the floor *plus* the stiffness results in a whole body movement that is a fine tremble or "jiggle," mostly in the vertical dimension.

Weakness of the Hip Girdle, Lower Back, and Abdominal Muscles

This type of abnormal gait is usually a result of muscular dystrophy, although myositis, poliomyelitis, and amyotrophic lateral sclerosis may be causes.

The patient "waddles" from side to side and has a protuberant abdomen, increased lumbar lordosis, and great difficulty in getting up from a chair.

Gait Apraxia

Gait apraxia is almost always of gradual onset and is slowly progressive. In its early form the patient walks with her feet close together, takes small steps (each step being less than the length of her foot), and walks with her hips and knees flexed. There are frequent pauses followed by another series of small steps.

The gait deteriorates over months or years until the patient cannot walk at all. An attendant on either side of her or a mechanical walker in front of her makes no difference. Her feet appear *glued* to the floor. If you move one of her feet out in front of her at the usual distance of a normal stride and ask her to bring the other foot forward, she will inch it forward in multiple small slides up to, but not in front of, the formerly forward foot.

The obscurity of the disorder is compounded when, on examination, you find the normal restless movements of the feet and see the patient cross and uncross her legs in a normal way while sitting. There are no signs of upper motor neuron, sensory system, basal ganglion, or cerebellar disease. These patients can mimic normal walking movements or mimic pedaling a bicycle while lying supine on the examining table.

This gait disorder may be associated with dementia and frontal lobe signs. However, often the association is not present and many severely demented patients have normal gait.

Normal-Pressure Hydrocephalus

The symptom triad suggesting normal-pressure hydrocephalus is dementia, gait ataxia, and urinary incontinence. However, all these symptoms need not be present and need not be equally severe. The ataxia, when present, may be wide-based, slow, awkward walking. It is not the same in each patient with the disease and sometimes resembles the gait apraxia described in the previous section.

Other Diseases to Consider When the Patient Is Ataxic

- Friedreich's ataxia
- Hereditary cerebellar ataxia
- Olivopontocerebellar degeneration
- Cerebellar ataxia with conjunctival telangiectasia
- Parenchymatous cerebellar degeneration—As a nutritional disorder in chronic alcoholics or as a remote nonmetastatic manifestation of carcinoma
- Increased intracranial pressure
- Overdose of many different drugs

Reflexes   13

This chapter describes three types of reflexes:

- Tendon or muscle stretch reflexes
- Superficial reflexes
- Primitive reflexes

Reflexes are an important part of the neurological examination and require some, but minimal, cooperation from the patient. They are *objective* evidence of the state of the nervous system.

TENDON OR MUSCLE STRETCH REFLEXES

Examination of a tendon reflex is the examination of the **reflex arc** and a number of **suprasegmental systems** that inhibit, condition, and modify the quality of the reflex.

The segmental reflex arc is made up of an afferent and efferent system. The afferent system has its cells in the posterior root ganglion, and its receptors are the muscle spindles and Golgi tendon organ. The arc is monosynaptic, and the efferent fibers arise from the anterior horn cells. There are both gamma (to the muscle spindles) and alpha (to the motor end plates) efferent fibers, and both are governed by suprasegmental systems.

Some people have no tendon reflexes anywhere. A *single* absent tendon reflex (except for the jaw jerk) is an abnormal reflex. The disease is in the arc and is most commonly in the nerve or root. Diseases of muscle, nerve, root, or cord can abolish the tendon reflex.

Tendon reflexes in the lower limbs are easier to elicit and more active than those in the upper limbs. Patients who are young, excitable, or embarrassed often have more active tendon reflexes.

The bounds of just what is a normal or abnormal tendon reflex are not precisely defined. We often have to decide by evaluating other accompanying physical signs and comparing the reflexes on the left half of the body with those on the right or the reflexes in the upper limbs with those in the lower limbs.

When a tendon reflex is abnormal (other than being absent), the following synonymous terms are used to describe it: *brisk, hyperactive, increased*, or *pathological*. An abnormal tendon reflex is never *faster* than a normal reflex. (It looks faster, but it is not. It can become slower, but never faster than normal.)

The only guidelines to help identify an *abnormal* or increased tendon reflex are as follows:

1. The **stimulus threshold**: Is the amount of force used to stretch the tendon and evoke a contraction less than experience suggests is normal, or less than is needed to evoke a response from the same reflex on the other side of the body? If the same forceful muscle contraction is elicited when using the handle of the reflex hammer on your middle finger instead of the head of the hammer, then the stimulus threshold is decreased and the reflex is increased and abnormal.
2. The **reflexogenic zone**: How big is the area from which the knee reflex may be elicited? Usually, it is the patellar tendon only. If the reflex is evoked by striking the middle of the tibia, then the reflexogenic zone is increased and the reflex is abnormal. This is another manifestation of reduced stimulus threshold.
3. The **extent and duration of the response**: Normally, only the quadriceps contracts in response to patellar tendon stretching and not *all* of the quadriceps. In an abnormal reflex more of the muscle contracts, it lasts longer, and other muscles (adductors or even the opposite quadriceps) may also contract. A normal knee reflex might be visible contraction of the quadriceps and no movement of the leg. The abnormal knee reflex might consist of extension of the knee to a straight leg position and a slow relaxation.

Summary

Diseases of the segmental reflex arc abolish tendon reflexes; diseases of the suprasegmental system enhance them.

The following reflexes are examined routinely. They are described with the patient lying down. It is helpful if the patient is relaxed and the limbs are supported. Anxiety can increase tendon reflexes, but anxiety and contraction of the antagonists can also abolish a reflex. Use a reflex hammer with a *soft* head and enough weight to be effective. Do not poke. Use the hammer like a golf club with a swing-through motion.

Jaw Jerk

Fifth Cranial Nerve: Masseter Muscles

As shown in Figure 13–1, put your left index finger horizontally on the patient's chin. Strike your finger when the patient has her mouth *open* about 2 cm. Bring the hammer from above downward in the direction of the arrow.

An *abnormal* response is prompt closure of the jaw. Most people have no response. Therefore, the reflex has no value in the diagnosis of segmental lesions.

A unilateral suprasegmental lesion does not produce an abnormal jaw jerk; a bilateral lesion does.

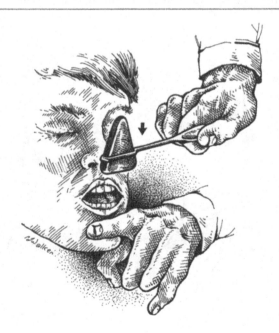

Figure 13–1. Jaw jerk is elicited by striking your own finger on the patient's chin while the patient's mouth is slightly open. The hammer motion is from above downward (arrow).

Biceps Reflex

Musculocutaneous Nerve: Sixth Cervical Root, Biceps and Brachialis Muscles The patient should be supine with his arms at his sides and his elbows flexed to 30–45 degrees. His arms are supine.

Stand on the right side of the examining table to examine the right biceps reflex. Put your left index and middle fingers on the biceps tendon as shown in Figure 13–2A. Push your fingers into the antecubital fossa and partially supinate your hand, stretching the skin in the antecubital fossa. This lengthens the biceps tendon and puts it very slightly on the stretch. Then hit your fingers with the hammer. Keep the direction of the hammer head parallel to the long axis of the biceps muscle as in Figure 13–2B.

A normal response is contraction of the biceps muscle, usually not strong enough to cause forearm flexion. With a suprasegmental lesion other muscles (eg, finger flexors or brachioradialis) may contract and there may be a greater contraction of the biceps, often causing forearm flexion. With a segmental le-

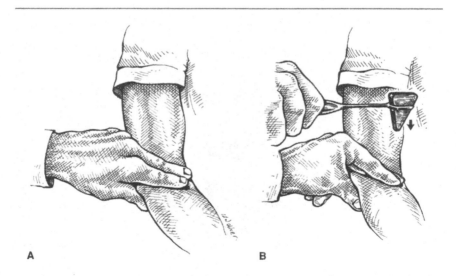

A   B

Figure 13–2. Examination of the biceps reflex. **A.** The examiner's fingers stretch the biceps tendon. **B.** The examiner supinates his own fingers into the antecubital fossa, further stretching the tendon. Keep the hammer direction parallel to the long axis of the biceps muscle.

sion (C6 root) the biceps will not contract, but small contractions of the finger flexors may be seen. This is known as inversion of the biceps reflex.

Supinator or Brachialis Reflex

Radial Nerve: Sixth Cervical Root, Brachioradialis Muscle

> The patient is in the same position as for the biceps reflex except that her forearm is midway between prone and supine. Strike the radius just proximal to its styloid process.

A normal response is a visible and palpable contraction of the brachioradialis muscle, usually not sufficiently strong to flex the forearm. With a suprasegmental lesion the response is abnormal as described above, and with a C6 segmental lesion the brachioradialis does not contract but the finger flexors will (ie, an inverted supinator reflex).

Triceps Reflex

Radial Nerve: Seventh and Eighth Cervical Roots, Triceps Muscle

> The patient should be supine. Stand on his right to examine the left triceps reflex. Place his left forearm across his abdomen, supported by his body, and his elbow at about a right angle. Gently pull his left hand toward you and strike the triceps tendon.

The normal response is less than the response of the biceps reflex and does not cause extension of the forearm.

If the reflex cannot be obtained, alter the degree of flexion at the elbow and use reinforcement (see the section on "Reinforcement," later in this chapter).

Finger Flexion Reflex

The finger flexion reflex has no diagnostic value at the segmental level. It is absent in many people. The reflex is informative, however, when it is present in one arm but not the other.

> Hold the patient's hand by the fingers as in Figure 13–3A. Produce a little extension at the patient's wrist and flexion at both his metacarpophalangeal and interphalangeal joints. Ask him to rest the weight of his arm and hand in your hand. Then gently tap the dorsum of your fingers with the reflex hammer. The patient's fingers flex as they gently grasp your fingers.

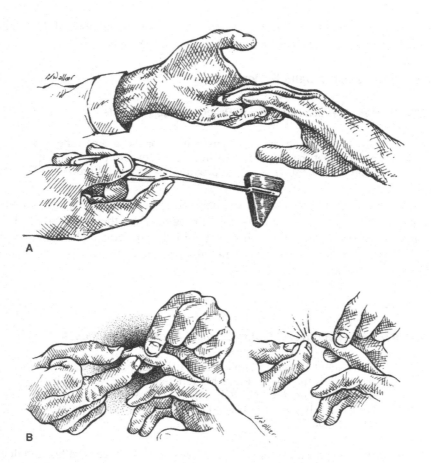

Figure 13–3. A. To assess finger flexion tone, the patient's left hand is held in the examiner's left hand. The examiner strikes the dorsum of his own fingers with the hammer. **B.** The Hoffmann reflex. The method is described in the text.

If present in both hands, the reflex means nothing. After you have done this several hundred times, you may be able to reliably identify an increased finger flexion response as abnormal. When it is present on one side but not the other, this is strong evidence that there is a suprasegmental lesion pertaining to the limb with the finger flexion.

Hoffmann's Reflex

Hoffmann's reflex is also of no diagnostic value at the segmental level. It is absent in most people. However, this is another way to assess the tone in the finger flexors and is most useful when it is present on one side but not the other.

Hold the sides of the patient's middle finger at the distal interphalangeal joint between your thumb and index finger as in Figure 13–3B. Forcefully and quickly flex the patient's middle finger distal phalanx, and immediately let go so that the phalanx pops into extension.

This will stretch the profundus flexor of the patient's middle finger. It and the other finger and thumb flexors will then contract if their tone is increased.

Knee Reflex

Femoral Nerve: Third and Fourth Lumbar Roots, Quadriceps Muscle

With the patient supine (or sitting), always flex the knee to about a right angle. If the patient is supine, support his knee with your hand or a pillow. As you compare the right and left knee reflexes, make sure the amount of knee flexion (and therefore quadriceps stretching) is the same in the two legs. Strike the patellar tendon.

A normal response varies from a flicker of visible contraction of the quadriceps to extension of the leg, lifting the foot off the bed or table.

Ankle Reflex

Tibial Nerve: First Sacral Root, Gastrocnemius and Soleus Muscles There are several methods to elicit this reflex. Unfortunately, the most convenient and quickest are the least sensitive and least reliable.

- As in Figure 13–4A, with the patient supine and his legs extended at the knee, place the dorsum of your hand gently on the sole of the patient's foot and passively dorsiflex the foot. Then strike the palm of your hand with the hammer. You have used the foot as a lever to stretch the Achilles tendon and the gastrocnemius and soleus muscles. If there is no muscle contraction by this method, this does *not* mean that the reflex is absent; try the following method.
- As in Figure 13–4B (this is the conventional method), place one foot on the opposite shin, thereby flexing the knee. Apply gentle pressure to dorsiflex the foot and then strike the tendon. If there is no response try the following. (Note: When the patient was *prone* and strength in the hamstrings and gluteus maximus muscles was being tested, there was an opportunity to examine the ankle reflex.)

- Flex the knee as in Figure 13–4C. Put gentle pressure on the sole of the foot to evoke some dorsiflexion and muscle stretching, then strike the tendon. If the reflex is absent by this method, there is disease in the segmental arc.
- Having the patient kneel on the edge of the examining table with his back to you is about as reliable as the previous method. As in Figure 13–4D, passively dorsiflex the foot before you strike the tendon.

Clonus

Clonus has the same significance as pathological tendon stretch reflexes, which were defined at the start of this section (ie, it is almost always indicative of suprasegmental disease).

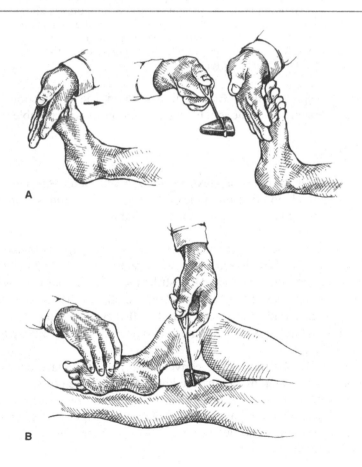

A

B

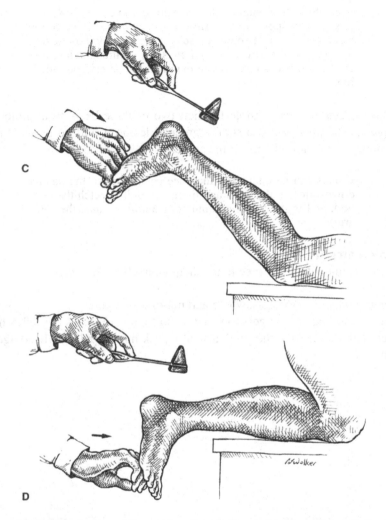

Figure 13–4. Examination of the ankle reflex. **A.** The patient is supine with the knee extended. The examiner gently dorsiflexes the patient's foot (arrow) and then strikes his own fingers with the hammer. **B.** A more sensitive method of examining the reflex. The examiner passively dorsiflexes the foot. **C.** Probably the best method of assessing the ankle reflex. The examiner dorsiflexes the foot (arrow). **D.** Similar to C. The patient kneels on the examining table, then the examiner passively dorsiflexes the foot (arrow) and strikes the tendon.

With the patient supine, flex his hip and knee to 30–45 degrees. Then apply *sudden, sustained, gentle* stretching to the gastrocnemius and soleus muscles by passively dorsiflexing the foot. These stretched calf muscles contract, relax, and contract again as long as you maintain the passive dorsiflexion.

This is **clonus**. It is possible to elicit two or three beats from almost all people. In the presence of a suprasegmental lesion it will go on as long as you maintain the dorsiflexion at the ankle.

Clonus can be elicited at the knee (rapidly push the patella downward), in the wrist and fingers (rapidly stretch the flexors), and in the forearm supinator (rapidly pronate the forearm).

Reinforcement

If you cannot elicit the knee reflex, help yourself as follows:

- Tell the patient to look elsewhere and not to watch you.
- Tell him to hook his fingers together, as in Figure 13–5. As the reflex hammer is about to strike the patellar tendon, ask him to pull one hand against the other.

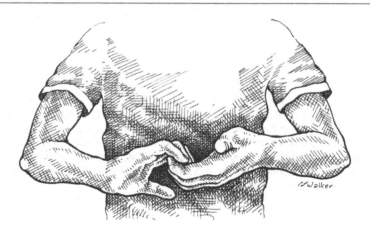

Figure 13–5. Reinforcement of the tendon reflexes. As the examiner strikes the tendon, the patient is asked to pull.

- If you cannot obtain an arm reflex, ask the patient to curl the fingers of the other hand into a loose fist. As you are about to deliver with the reflex hammer, ask him to make a tight, strong fist.

SUPERFICIAL REFLEXES

Corneal Reflex
Examination of the corneal reflex reveals information about the segmental reflex arc and the suprasegmental system as high as the contralateral thalamus. (See the section on the fifth cranial nerve in Chapter 8.)

Pharyngeal Reflex
The pharyngeal reflex is often absent. (See the sections on the ninth and tenth cranial nerves in Chapter 9.)

Abdominal Reflexes
Like the corneal reflex, the abdominal reflexes may be abolished by ipsilateral segmental or contralateral suprasegmental lesions. The stimulus is pain or touch, and the response is a simple abdominal muscle contraction.

> The patient must be supine and relaxed. Stroke the skin of the abdomen with a pin, pencil, or the pointed handle of the reflex hammer, in the direction of the arrows shown in Figure 13–6. Keep each stimulus within the approximate dermatome of an individual spinal nerve. Move the stimulus toward the midline each time. The normal response is contraction of the underlying muscle and movement of the umbilicus toward the stimulus. Do *not* make the stimulus so strong that it stretches the underlying muscle directly. The stimulus is applied to the *skin*.

Lesions of spinal nerves or roots from T7 to T11 will abolish the reflexes.

The abdominal reflex is dependent on the integrity of a multisynaptic suprasegmental system, part of which is the pyramidal tract. Thus, unilateral absent abdominal reflexes can be an early and sensitive sign of recent acute pyramidal tract disease.

Abdominal reflexes are usually absent in patients with lax, stretched abdominal muscles and in the elderly.

Cremasteric Reflex

> Stroke the inner upper aspect of the thigh with a pin or pencil. The stimulus is of the same quality as was used to elicit

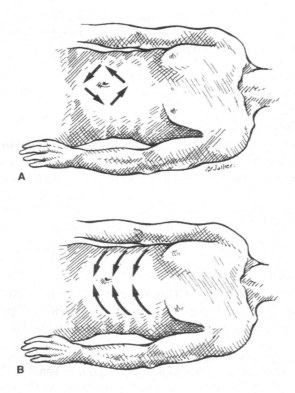

Figure 13–6. Abdominal reflexes should be obtained by moving the stimulus in the direction of the arrows as in **B,** not as in **A.**

the abdominal reflexes. A response is elevation of the testicle (not the scrotum) on the same side.

The reflex will be abolished with segmental lesions of the first and second lumbar roots or cord segments and, like the abdominal reflex, in lesions of the corticospinal tract.

Plantar Reflex

The **extensor** plantar response is a sensitive, early, reliable sign of corticospinal tract disease. It has no localizing value, however, when the patient is in a coma for any reason or asleep. It has no diagnostic usefulness as a sign of segmental disease. Stroking the sole of the foot of most people results in rapid hip and knee flexion, dorsiflexion at the ankle, and plantar flexion and adduction of the toes. It is important that you watch this series of movements in every patient that you examine.

The normal response is called a **flexor plantar response**. The abnormal response is *extension* of the big toe and *abduction* of the other toes. This is the **extensor plantar response**, or Babinski response. The important thing to watch is the *big toe*.

- The lower limb should be extended at the hip and knee (ie, with the patient fully supine).
- The stimulus should be firm and noxious.
- Stroke the sole of the foot with the blunt handle of the reflex hammer.
- Start at the heel on the lateral aspect and move the stimulus toward the toes.

Stop the stimulus when a response is obtained. The big toe may extend after the stimulus has moved 3 cm or less. The total movement of the stimulus can be up the lateral edge of the foot to the little toe and then across the sole to the head of the metatarsal of the big toe. The *response* has usually appeared before the stimulus has moved this far.

If the patient will not let you touch the sole of her foot, you may apply the afferent stimulus at

- The posterolateral aspect of the foot, as a stroking motion from behind and below the lateral malleolus, continuing it up the dorsolateral *edge* of the foot
- The edge of the tibia, by pressing on the bone at the tuberosity and running your fingers firmly down the length of the shin to the ankle
- The calf, by squeezing the gastrocnemius and soleus muscles

All of these are less reliable methods than applying the stimulus to the sole of the foot.

Primitive Reflexes

All of the primitive reflexes are present in healthy babies and are innate. They disappear, however, as the higher cerebral centers develop with maturity. They may reappear with disease or damage to these centers.

Grasp Reflex

The grasp reflex may be present bilaterally in patients who are semiconscious or fully alert. Like the extensor plantar response in the same clinical setting, this is not very useful information.

> Put your index and middle fingers or the handle of the reflex hammer on the palm of the patient's hand and slowly stroke the palm toward the thumb or little finger.

The patient's fingers flex and grasp the handle of the hammer. If you are quick, you can remove the stimulus before it is caught. Sometimes a simple nonmoving touch to the patient's palm will evoke finger flexion. You may repeat the stimulus indefinitely and provoke finger flexion each time. Tell the patient "Do not squeeze this [handle] when I put it in your hand"—he can overcome the reflex and not do it, usually *once only*. Once he has grasped it, he usually cannot open his hand on command.

This reflex indicates contralateral frontal lobe disease. The reflex will vanish in the presence of corticospinal tract disease.

Sucking Reflex

Ask the patient to open his mouth 2 cm, then touch his lips with a wet tongue blade, moving the stick from the lateral aspect of the lips to the midline and then laterally again.

The response is a sucking motion of the upper and lower lips.

The response can also be obtained by gently tapping the upper or lower lip with the reflex hammer.

This reflex also indicates frontal lobe disease. It is also present, however, when there is a bilateral corticospinal tract lesion above the midpons.

Palmar-Mental Reflex

Scratch the patient's palm with the handle of the reflex hammer. The scratch should be firm and the direction should be from the fingers to the wrist or vice versa. A positive response is a short-duration flicker or dimple in the skin of the chin. This indicates contralateral frontal lobe disease; it will vanish after a corticospinal tract lesion and its veracity and usefulness are not proven.

Sensation **14**

This part of the examination is difficult, and findings are not always reproducible. The tests are crude, and the results are dependent on the cooperation of and interpretation by the patient.

Sensory findings are always *subjective*. A painless ulcer on the sole of an anesthetic foot or a cigarette burn on the edge of the middle finger are objective signs, but their significance rests on what the patient *says* about them.

Sensory symptoms depend on the vocabulary and intelligence of the patient. Descriptions such as "numb," "tingling," "prickling," "asleep," and "like dental anesthetic coming out" are the most common. The rare patient says "The part is dead; there is no feeling in it at all." Others say that the part (eg, the side of the face) is normal or unremarkable if it is not touched but feels different when he shaves, for example.

More subtle sensory symptoms are descriptions such as "My fingers [or toes] feel swollen like sausages," "The skin is too tight," or "I feel as though I have tight gloves on all the time."

Symptoms in the lower limbs may be described in this way: "I feel as though I'm walking on cotton wool" (possibly a posterior column lesion) or "My shoes are full of small stones; my feet are on fire" (a possible peripheral nerve lesion) as well as the more usual descriptions of numbness, tingling, and prickling. The **proximal pain and peripheral paresthesia** clue—"I have pain in my shoulder and down the back beside my shoulder blade and my little finger is asleep"—clearly tells you where the sensory signs should be.

When you hear these symptoms, examine the part in more detail and, if necessary, examine only the symptomatic area the next day.

The patient with no sensory complaints (including pain) and nothing in his history to suggest a disturbance of sensation should have a sensory examination lasting 5 min, consisting of the following:

- Touch and pain sensation over the face (always the corneas), hands, feet, and trunk
- Vibration sense and joint passive movement sense in the fingers and toes

Rules of Sensory Examination

Fatigue Do not perform a sensory examination at the end of a lengthy examination process; the more tired the patient is, the more dubious the answers. Reliable signs are more likely when the sensory system is examined alone.

Suggestion Do not interfere with the patient's decisions by slanting your instructions toward the *abnormal.* When you are comparing pinprick on the two sides, say, "Does this [testing the right side] feel the *same* as this [testing the left side]?" Do not ask the patient if the two sides feel *different.*

Demonstration *Demonstrate* first what you are going to do. Touch the patient gently with the cotton several times in an area you *know* has normal sensation before you examine the area of concern. Say to him, "Each time you feel a touch, will you please say 'yes.' "

Put the vibrating tuning fork in the middle of the patient's sternum and tell him that it is the *vibration*—not the sound of the tuning fork or the pressure of the handle—you are concerned with.

Brevity *Brief* instructions, *brief* answers, and *brief* examinations are advised.

Keep your instructions simple. Ask the patient to answer *quickly* "yes" for each touch and "sharp" or "dull" when you touch him with the point or head of the pin. You do not want a qualified answer.

Eyes Closed Do not let the patient watch you do the sensory examination. Have your assistant or the patient hold up the bedsheet to cut off the patient's vision from the part being examined. If the examination is brief and limited (eg, the sensory disturbance is a median nerve lesion at the wrist), you can ask him to close his eyes.

Dementia, Delirium, and Confusional States Patients in any of these categories cannot be examined for sensation except in the most crude way, such as corneal reflexes or withdrawal of the limb from repetitive pinprick.

Examine from the Abnormal to the Normal The patient with numb weak legs should have his sensory level established by being examined from below upward. The pin can be moved in short quick steps or more slowly dragged over the skin.

Medicolegal Litigation Patients who have been in accidents or who have been injured at work or where a third party is involved require special mention. If they have sensory findings, draw a map of the limb or body part involved and shade in the area of abnormality. Use slash marks for pain loss, dots for touch loss, and so on. Draw the map immediately after the examination.

Definitions

Analgesia: Loss of appreciation of pain sensation

Anesthesia: Loss of appreciation of all forms of sensation

Dysesthesia: An unpleasant and abnormal response to an innocuous stimulus

Hypalgesia: Decreased appreciation of pain sensation

Hyperesthesia: Abnormally increased sensitivity to any stimulus

Hyperpathia: Abnormally increased sensitivity to a pain stimulus

Hypoesthesia: Decreased appreciation of all forms of sensation

Paresthesia: An abnormal, spontaneous sensation (eg, tingling or crawling)

TOUCH

The test object for touch is usually a piece of cotton wool. Pull the fibers out so that you are using only a small amount of the cotton. Shield the patient's vision. Tell him what you are going to do—touch him—and tell him that each time you do this he should say "yes." The force of the touch should not deform the skin. A touch does not mean drag or wipe the cotton over the skin. This is tickling and is anatomically related to pain conduction. A touch is an end-point touch.

On most faces, 10 touches will result in 10 answers. On other parts of the body some touches are normally ignored, but usually not more than one or two out of 20. Is the number of ignored touches the same on the two halves of the body? Hairy parts of the body are exquisitely sensitive to touch stimulation. Bending a hair by touching it stimulates both superficial and deep sensory systems. Lack of response to a touched hair is never normal.

Hallucinatory Answers

Apply the stimulus in an irregular rhythm so the patient does not anticipate it. Sometimes, after a pause of 5 s, during which *no* stimulus has been applied, the patient says "yes." This may represent a conduction delay in which he is responding to the last touch. Usually, however, it is not. When these "spontaneous" or hallucinatory responses occur as often on the right half of the body as on the left, or as often from the normal areas as from the symptomatic region, they are not diagnostic.

If responses occur on stimulation of one limb only or on one half of the body only, that area is usually the abnormal one.

An occasional litigious patient with a numb arm will say "yes" to 95% of the touches over all of his body except the arm. Each time you touch the arm, he says "no." This tells you two things about him. First, he is not thinking; second, his numbness is not organic.

Lesions

With **peripheral nerve lesions** the area of touch loss is greater than the area of pain loss.

With **spinal cord lesions** if there is a *loss* of touch sensation, the patient usually cannot walk. Touch is conveyed by several tracts in the cord.

With **parietal lobe lesions** many touches will not be perceived, while others of the same intensity in the same area will be and there will be frequent hallucinatory responses.

The most sensitive test of touch is in localization. Before touch sense is absent, the patient will be unable to accurately locate the touched area. For this reason the cotton used should be a few small, teased threads only.

SUPERFICIAL PAIN

The common testing object for superficial pain is a pin. Use a sterile common pin, which you will discard at the end of the examination. Tell the patient that you do not always do this with exactly the same amount of pressure each time.

Touch the point of the pin to some part of the patient's skin where you know sensation is normal. Tell him that this is "sharp." Touch the head on the other end of the pin to the same area and tell him that this is "dull." Then test the patient's pain perception on his face, hands and feet, arms, legs, and trunk. The cornified skin on the normal palm and sole are not highly sensitive to pain.

Test a large area, not a small spot. Repetitive stimuli on the same hypoesthetic spot may be felt as sharp or sharper than normal. Repetitive stimuli are cumulative and can overcome an elevated pain threshold. "Pain spots" perceive the pin more acutely, and some touches with the pin will hit them. Other areas are relatively insensitive, with fewer pain spots. Therefore, keep the pin moving and use the point and the head with equal frequency, comparing the responses from a large area on one side to the responses from the homologous area on the other side of the body.

If you find an abnormal area, are other sensations abnormal here as well? Does the area conform to a spinal or peripheral *nerve* distribution? Does it have a spinal *cord* configuration, and if so, is there a level? Is it present in the homologous area of the trunk or limb of the opposite side?

Pain perception may be **delayed**. This is abnormal. Touch the dorsum of the foot and ask the patient to say "yes" as soon as she feels it. She should answer almost before you have lifted the pin from the skin.

Faulty pain localization is particularly useful in the diagnosis of cerebral lesions. With the patient's eyes closed, touch her with the pin and ask her to point to the spot with one finger. This is normally more accurate in the distal than in the proximal part of the limbs.

Hallucinatory responses occur with pain testing. They are of the same significance as this type of response with touch testing.

Pain is **cumulative**. The last part of the body to be tested perceives the identical pinprick more acutely than the first part tested. Therefore, reverse the order of testing if this might explain why the patient says the last part tested was more sensitive.

TEMPERATURE

Use large (250-mm-long) test tubes with rubber stoppers. Cold tap water at about 20° C and hot water at about 45° C provide an adequate difference to start.

Keep the outside of the tubes dry. There is no feeling of wetness, but a wet tube is interpreted as a cold tube.

Apply the side of the tube, not the small bottom, to the skin. This sensation should be tested *slowly*. There is a normal longer latency between application of the thermal stimulus and the response than with pain or touch stimulation. Let the hot or cold tube, especially the hot one, stay on the skin for 2 s each time.

If the patient has paresthesias and testing for touch and pain yields normal results, sometimes temperature testing gives useful information.

The purpose is to see whether the hot and cold tubes are *as hot* or *as cold* in the area of concern as in a normal area. Once it has been established that there is an area less sensitive than the normal area, the ability to differentiate within that area may be defined by reducing the temperature difference in the two tubes. When the water in the tube is about 30° C, the normal person can differentiate a 1° difference in temperature. Slowly sliding the hot tube over the skin (from abnormal to normal) will often define the boundaries of an area of decreased sensation.

Expose the area to be examined to room temperature for 15 min before starting. Reliable answers cannot be obtained from skin areas that are cold and vasoconstricted.

Remember: Contact the skin with a large area of the tube for at least 2 s per stimulus.

DEEP PAIN

Deep pain sensation may be intact even when the response to pinprick is abnormal. The stimulus is squeezing the Achilles tendon or the calf or biceps muscle. The normal response is an uncomfortable deep, slow, poorly localized pain accompanied by nausea and protestations from the patient.

VIBRATION SENSE

Use a tuning fork that vibrates at 128 per second. A normal adult can feel a vigorously vibrating tuning fork for 12–15 s at the ankle and for 15–20 s on the distal phalanx of the index finger.

Instruct the patient as you place the handle of the vibrating fork on his sternum or jaw. Tell him you want to know when the vibration stops. Demonstrate this by grasping the vibrating tines of the fork with your other hand while the handle is firmly against his sternum. This will stop the vibration.

Make the tuning fork vibrate by hitting it close to the base of the tines with the heel of your hand. Put the handle on a distal bony prominence (eg, the big toe or either malleolus at the ankle; if there is no sense of vibration, you must move to a more proximal bony point). Ask the patient to tell you when the vibration stops. Let the tuning fork "run down" on its own.

When the patient says that the vibrating has stopped at the right medial malleolus, if you then quickly put the handle on the left medial malleolus (without striking the fork again) the vibration is felt again for a few seconds. In spite of what is stated in some textbooks, this is *normal*.

The decrease in vibratory sense may be gradual, being absent at the big toe and ankle and felt for 2–3 s at the knee, 5 s at the iliac spine, and 15 s over the spinous process of the first lumbar vertebra. These findings are consistent with a peripheral nerve lesion *or* a degenerative disease of the posterior columns of the spinal cord.

If vibratory sense is absent at the ankle, knee, and pelvis and normal at some spinous process, this is consistent with a transverse, compressive, or destructive lesion of the spinal cord.

Vibratory sense and passive joint movements are each served by different portions of the posterior columns of the spinal cord and may not be equally abnormal. Apparently, otherwise normal older people have decreased or absent vibration sense at the ankles because of a segmental peripheral neuropathy of unknown cause. Subacute combined degeneration of the spinal cord is marked by a greater vibratory loss than passive joint movement loss. Tabes dorsalis is the reverse. Vibratory sense is not impaired in cerebral lesions above the thalamus, while defective sense of passive movement in one big toe may be a critical physical sign of the parasagittal, parietal meningioma (ie, it is a cortical sensation).

SENSE OF PASSIVE MOVEMENT

Ask the patient to watch you. If the patient does not receive a proper demonstration and instructions before you start this test, the response may be wrong half the time. Passive movement is tested at one joint only, starting at the most distal toe or finger. Hold the proximal phalanx of the patient's big toe in your left hand and anchor it. Grasp the *sides* of the distal phalanx of the big toe between your right thumb and index finger. Move the distal phalanx of the toe slowly up (dorsiflexion) a random number of times, telling the patient that each of these movement is "up." Do the same thing while moving the toe down. Then, with his vision shielded, make random up-and-down movements (eg, three up, two down, one up, four down), asking him to tell you each time where it is. A wrong answer for the first move in a new direction is normal. Move the distal phalanx slowly, consistently, and a small distance each time.

POSITION SENSE

Does the patient know where his limbs are in space? A defect of this sensation produces a major disability. With the patient sitting, his eyes closed, and an arm held out in front of him (see Figure 10–1), an arm with defective position sense will drift. This limb will often have slow, continuing, restless movements called pseudoathetosis.

With the patient's eyes closed, move the abnormal limb several times and ask him to point to it with the other (normal) index finger. Place the abnormal limb in a certain position and ask the patient, with his eyes closed, to imitate the position with his normal limb. If position sense is defective, he cannot do either. This sensation is defective in diseases of the posterior root, posterior columns, and parietal lobe.

STEREOGNOSIS

Stereognosis can be assessed only when touch, pain, temperature, and vibration sense in the hand are all *normal*. Can the patient, with his eyes closed, identify common objects placed in his hand? He must be capable of *moving* the object in his hand and quickly feeling it with his fingers and thumb. A paralyzed hand cannot be examined for stereognosis. Use a key, coin, pocketknife, and pen. All the objects, or all but one, may be identified correctly after 15–20 s of examination in one hand and in the other after 3 s. The former is abnormal. If the objects are not identified in either hand but are recognized visually, only one lesion is present; the patient has tactile agnosia but not astereognosis.

NUMBER WRITING

Number writing is also a test of cortical sensory integration. "Write" on the patient's palm random, single-digit numbers, first with her watching you, then with her eyes closed. The bigger the drawing and the firmer and faster the movement of the pencil, the easier it is for her to correctly guess the number.

TWO-POINT DISCRIMINATION

The ability to tell one from two touches that are close together may be defective in lesions of peripheral nerves, the posterior columns of the spinal cord, and the cerebrum. A pair of dividers with dull points or an unwound wire paper clip can be used to test this sensation.

The normal threshold on the lip is probably 1 mm, on the tip of the index finger is 3–5 mm, and on the back is several centimeters. The two points of the dividers are placed on the skin simultaneously with equal pressure. If the sensation is defective in the index finger, two points at 5-mm separation will be felt as one and may still be one at 9- to 10-mm separation, while the opposite (normal) side can identify two points at a separation of 3 mm. Some single-point touches on the abnormal side will also be interpreted as two.

BILATERAL SIMULTANEOUS STIMULATION

Sensory neglect of one half of the body or of one limb may be an isolated sensory finding or part of a constellation of cerebral sensory signs.

If the patient has a right parietal lesion, for example, the sensory examination of his left side may be uninformative. However, if you touch the identical spot on the back of his right and left hands with cotton at the same moment and ask him, while his eyes are closed, to tell you where he has been touched, he will consistently say "right"; that is, when stimulated simultaneously, he ignores the *left* side. When you touch his left side *only*, he always says "left." Similarly, touching the right side *only* always provokes a correct answer. Sensory neglect revealed by bilateral simultaneous stimulation may be the only or the earliest sensory abnormality.

SUMMARY

All bedside sensory findings are subjective except the corneal reflex. Remember:

- Sensory examination should be of brief duration, with brief instructions, and brief answers.
- In peripheral nerve lesions touch and superficial pain are most likely to be abnormal.
- In posterior root lesions position sense, passive movement, and, to a lesser extent, vibration sense will be abnormal.
- In spinal cord disease superficial pain and temperature, sense of passive movement, and vibration will be affected, depending on what area of the cord is diseased, with relative preservation of touch. When touch is lost because of cord disease, the patient usually cannot walk.
- In parietal lobe lesions discriminatory sensations are abnormal. These are: sense of passive movement, number writing, two-point discrimination, stereognosis, tactile or pain localization, and the recognition of two simultaneous stimuli on homologous body parts. It is not possible to say which of these is most likely to be abnormal in any particular lesion.

The Cerebellum 15

The signs of cerebellar disease are more obvious when the lesion is unilateral and disease in other parts of the nervous system is absent. The signs vary, depending on whether the lesion is acute or chronic, bilateral or unilateral, and hemispheric or midline.

MUSCLE TONE

Cerebellar lesions reduce muscle tone. Diseases of the hemispheres or the vermis will produce hypotonia; with the latter, it will be more manifest in the trunk.

The hypotonia is ipsilateral to the side of the lesion and more marked when the lesion is acute. The affected limbs can be displaced into abnormal postures with less sense of resistance, joints are hyperextendable, and the range of limb movement is increased.

POSTURE

Cerebellar disease will cause the unsupported arm (held in front of the patient, with his eyes closed) to waiver and drift. It may be tremulous or may have irregular, purposeless, repetitive, **pseudoathetotic** movements. These are also seen when position sense is defective. While the patient holds the limb still, as in testing for arm drift, if you gently tap the wrist to either side, up or down, an abnormally large movement results. The same can be demonstrated in the lower limb.

TENDON REFLEXES

In acute cerebellar lesions such as hemorrhage or trauma, all the tendon reflexes may be absent for hours or days. After that they may be obtainable but temporarily depressed.

In the less acute lesion some tendon reflexes are **pendular**.

Ask the patient to sit well forward on the edge of the examining table. Strike the patellar tendon as usual.

The leg will extend at the knee, then flex, and then extend again three or four times, with a *decreasing* range each time. The braking action of the quadriceps antagonists (the hamstrings) does not dampen the response after the first contraction of the quadriceps.

Pendular reflexes are not an exclusive cerebellar sign and may be present in any hypotonic condition.

TREMOR

Cerebellar tremor is an action or intention tremor and disappears when the part is completely supported and at rest. It results from disease of the dentate nucleus or its connections. The stationary outstretched upper limbs may show a rhythmic constant tremor. This can be a flexion-extension tremor at the wrist at three or four per second or of the whole arm at the shoulder, somewhat slower and more coarse.

When the patient is sitting, a tremor of about the same frequency may involve the head. It is usually an affirmative nodding tremor and often has periodicity to it. There will be 10 or 12 beats with more or less regular synchrony, then a pause and no tremor for 5–10 s, and then the tremor resumes. The pause is often associated with a minor change in head position or perhaps the patient touched his chin or cheek with a finger. Often, however, the tremor appears to stop and start spontaneously. It will disappear when the patient is lying down and the head is fully supported.

The intention tremor of the unsupported, stationary upper limb becomes less regular and less obvious when the limb starts to move. As the patient brings the index finger from the fully outstretched position toward the tip of the nose, there is clearly an irregularity and jerkiness to the passage, but in the final few inches before the finger touches the nose the tremor will explode. It becomes faster and wilder, and the hand thrashes back and forth. Immediately when the index finger contacts the nose, the whole thing dampens down and the tremor is reduced entirely or by 90%. This burst of tremor at the end of a voluntary movement also is not an exclusive cerebellar sign.

REBOUND, PAST POINTING, AND DYSMETRIA

To elicit rebound, have the patient flex his elbow to less than a right angle. Resist him by pulling on the volar surface of his wrist to extend his forearm. Stop suddenly by withdrawing your hand.

A person with disease of the cerebellum cannot stop the released forearm and may hit himself. The ability to quickly stop the flexion when the extensor force is withdrawn is defective.

When the patient with cerebellar disease performs the rapid alternating movements described in Chapter 10, abnormalities may become evident. This is most useful when cerebellar tremor is minimal or absent. When the patient attempts to touch the tip of his nose with his index finger, the finger will stop before it gets to the nose. On the next attempt he will overshoot and hit his nose too forcefully. When he is making rapid repetitive pinches of the thumb and index finger or repetitive prone-supine-prone pats with his hand on his thigh, you will see and hear the abnormality. The movements are of uneven strength, speed, and frequency.

VOLUNTARY MOVEMENTS

With acute cerebellar disease there may be weakness and slowness of voluntary movements. The weakness is transient. There may also be slowness of relaxation of voluntary movement.

NYSTAGMUS

A large, unilateral cerebellar hemisphere lesion will provoke coarse, slow nystagmus on gaze to the side of the lesion and faster, finer nystagmus on gaze to the other side.

Upbeat nystagmus may be seen in lesions of the vermis of the cerebellum, although disease of other parts of the brain stem can cause this nystagmus.

Downbeat nystagmus is usually seen in diseases at the cervicomedullary junction, including cerebellar herniation, Arnold-Chiari malformation, and platybasia.

Ocular dysmetria is similar to past pointing or overshooting of the hand. The patient attempts to fix gaze and the eyes overshoot, correct, overshoot to a lesser extent in the opposite direction, and after several successively smaller movements in either direction, will fix on the desired object. These movements can be rotary or vertical. *Ocular dysmetria, ocular flutter,* and *opsoclonus* are terms that may be used interchangeably.

Disorders of gait in cerebellar disease have been covered in Chapter 12.

SPEECH

The scanning, staccato speech of cerebellar disease is also called an ataxic dysarthria. The patient's speech sounds like a sobbing child who is trying to talk after crying. The diaphragm rises in a series of irregular jerks, variable in speed and amplitude. Multisyllabic words are broken into individual syllables and "Methodist" comes out as "Meth," "o," "dist." In addition, words are slurred. There is lack of lip, tongue, and pharynx coordination as well as irregular air propulsion as a result of diaphragm ataxia.

Finally, it should be remembered that a unilateral frontal lobe lesion can produce contralateral arm and leg ataxia, weakness, and an action tremor. This **diametric, diagnostic dilemma** is rare, but it does occur.

The Corticospinal System 16

The most common abnormal signs encountered in neurological practice are those of disease of the corticospinal system.

This system has several more or less synonymous names: the upper motor neuron, pyramidal tract, and descending supraspinal pathway. The corticospinal system is not a single tract. It includes the fibers arising from the Betz cells in cortical area 4, the longest uninterrupted white matter tract in the nervous system. It also includes the fibers of the rubrospinal, reticulospinal, and vestibulospinal tracts as well as the effects of the basal ganglia and cerebellum and their multisynaptic connections on the motor system.

All of these components are concerned with the facilitation, inhibition, control, and modulation of movement. The sensory system is also an important and integral contributor to normal movement.

The signs of disease of the corticospinal system depend on the level and location of the lesion and the rate of its development and progression.

All upper motor neuron lesions have some features in common, although one may cause spasticity and slowness of voluntary movement without marked weakness, while another may produce hypotonia and profound paresis.

The signs of the disease of the system may be considered under the headings of power, tone, reflexes, and miscellaneous.

POWER

When the lesion is above the midpons, expect weakness in the contralateral face, arm, and leg.

In Chapters 8 and 9 on the seventh and eleventh cranial nerves, the weakness of the lower face with *relatively* normal upper face strength and the details of the shoulder shrug versus head turning strength were discussed.

> Watch the *speed* and *range* of movement of the corner of the mouth when the patient shows his teeth on command.

However dense the paresis of the lower face may be, *emotional* facial movements will usually be normal on the paretic side.

Jaw opening and chewing will be normal, while half the tongue will be transiently paretic and the tongue will point to the paretic side when protruded. Although a lesion may produce permanent face, arm, and leg paresis, the tongue weakness is usually transient. Palate and pharynx movements are not affected by *unilateral* corticospinal system lesions.

Weakness of the upper limb is variable in amount but consistent in distribution. It is most marked and *earliest* (in a progressive lesion) in the **extensors** and **abductors** of the fingers. Extensors of the wrist and forearm will be affected, and eventually so will flexors. The common quick assessment of upper limb strength—"Squeeze my fingers"—is particularly inappropriate. By the time the finger flexors are involved, the weakness can be diagnosed by the posture of the limb. Minimal upper limb weakness may appear as slowness and awkwardness in fine, discrete movements. The best tests to demonstrate this are the rapid alternating movements described in Chapter 10. The maximum upper limb weakness is permanent loss of all useful movement.

In the lower limb, early and minimal weakness is first seen in the **flexors** of the thigh and **dorsiflexors** of the foot and toes. Tripping over the edge of a carpet, a curb, or a stair riser is a common early symptom.

Depending on the age of the lesion (whether it is spinal or cerebral and, if the latter, the level), the paretic leg may assume a flexed or extended position.

Following resolution of acute intracerebral lesions, the leg almost always regains some power.

TONE

Increased tone from disease of the corticospinal system is usually called spasticity. Rigidity usually implies extrapyramidal disease.

With a unilateral corticospinal system lesion above the brain stem, there are no changes in tone evident in the head and neck.

In the upper limb the increased tone is in the flexors of the fingers, wrist, and elbow. It is greatest in the early part of stretching. It can be abolished temporarily by repeated stretches and will return after the muscle has been put at rest. The posture of the upper limb is the consequence of **flexor muscle spasticity** and **extensor muscle weakness**.

In the lower limb, spasticity is first and greatest in the quadriceps, gastrocnemius, and soleus. The footdrop posture is also a combined manifestation, the foot being *dropped* down by dorsiflexor weakness and *pulled* down by plantar flexor spasticity.

A hemiparesis resulting from a *cortical* lesion (a very rare occurrence) will be flaccid and will remain this way. Many acute intracranial and all acute spinal, corticospinal tract lesions present initially with flaccid weakness. In the latter case this is called spinal shock. After days or weeks the limbs become spastic. An acute lesion in one cerebellar hemisphere will present with a flaccid, ipsilateral weakness, ataxia, and often absent reflexes.

REFLEXES

Corticospinal system lesions increase tendon reflexes and abolish superficial reflexes. The qualities of an increased reflex are listed in Chapter 13. A unilateral corticospinal system lesion above the midpons will not produce a jaw jerk; a bilateral lesion will.

An *acute* right-sided corticospinal system lesion above the decussation of the pyramids or a left-sided lesion below the decussation but above the seventh dorsal cord segment will abolish the left abdominal reflexes. In more chronic diseases such as amyotrophic lateral sclerosis and cerebral palsy, the abdominal reflexes are usually retained in spite of obvious corticospinal system involvement. The cremasteric reflex will disappear if the appropriate corticospinal lesion is present.

The plantar response is the most evanescent and difficult sign of corticospinal system disease. Almost no one likes the sole of his foot to be touched, tickled, or stroked. The normal withdrawal at the hip and knee diverts the examiner's attention away from the toes. One may scratch a patient's foot only a limited number of times.

The hip and knee should be in full extension, and the first attempt to elicit the response is usually the best attempt.

A tired patient admitted late in the day may have easily obtained and clearly extensor plantar responses. The same patient, after a good night's sleep, examined by the same person, may have flexor responses the next morning.

The plantar response seems to lend itself to equivocation in the patient's records. The reflex is often recorded as 0 or with two arrows, one pointing up and the other down. Make a decision; the examination is not over until this is decided. An aphoristic view of the equivocal plantar response suggests that if you cannot decide whether it is up or down, it is probably down. This is correct more often than not.

MISCELLANEOUS

The gait of the patient with a corticospinal system lesion in the internal capsule is distinctive. The arm and fingers are flexed and adducted and the leg is circumducted in an arc at the hip, while the foot is plantar flexed and inverted. There is little, if any, knee flexion with each step.

The posture of the acute hemiparetic patient in bed is abnormal. He may be lying on his paretic arm and not be concerned; the leg will be extended and externally rotated at the hip. Even when supine, there is more plantar flexion at the ankle on the paretic side than on the normal side.

Clonus may be elicited at the ankle, knee, or wrist. The method is described in Chapter 13. It is never the *only* sign of corticospinal tract disease and is not a useful physical sign.

CONCLUSIONS

When diseased, this huge, complex system has simple signs: weakness, slowness, and clumsiness of purposeful movement; changes in muscle tone, stretch, and superficial reflexes; and the addition of new reflexes.

There is a quantitative relationship between only two of these signs. If muscle tone is increased, the tendon reflexes will be increased. This is always true, unless the muscle is so stretched that striking its tendon can stretch it no further. The opposite relationship is *not* true: tendon reflexes may be pathologically brisk, while muscle tone is normal.

A minimal corticospinal system syndrome might consist of unilateral absent abdominal reflexes or an extensor plantar response. A larger constellation might consist of flaccid weakness of the arm and leg, pathologically brisk tendon reflexes, normal superficial reflexes, and a flexor plantar response.

The signs vary and are unrelated to each other in a quantitative way, except as mentioned above. The variations are dependent on site, size, and rate of progress of the lesion. A proper examination includes verification of all the possible manifestations of a corticospinal system lesion.

PSEUDOBULBAR PALSY

Pseudobulbar palsy is caused by **bilateral corticobulbar** system disease above the brain stem—most commonly, bilateral strokes that have occurred at different times. As the lesion is not in the bulb but *above* it, a more accurate title might be suprabulbar palsy.

The signs of bulbar dysfunction are

• Dysphagia—These patients have trouble chewing and swallowing. Food falls out of the mouth while eating or enters the larynx without provoking

coughing or remains in the mouth between the cheek and the teeth for hours after a meal.
- Dysarthria—Speech lacks resonance and variation in tone. It sounds strangled and is usually high-pitched and weak.
- Jaw jerk, snout, and sucking reflexes are usually present.
- The tongue cannot protrude beyond the teeth by more than 1 in, and rapid alternating movements of the tongue are not possible.
- Emotional control is defective. Words, situations, and events that are not sad will provoke uncontrollable crying. These patients also may laugh inappropriately but I have never witnessed the latter.
- Some signs of bilateral hemiparesis are present in the limbs.

Higher Cortical Functions: *Intelligence and Memory* 17

The majority of patients seen by the neurologist do not require testing of intelligence. In the course of history taking the patient's memory and intelligence are revealed and this is often sufficient.

However, a more formal examination must be carried out in the following situations:

- Where the **symptoms are vague, circumstantial**, and attributed to someone else—for example, "She says [pointing to his wife] I keep losing my glasses and my keys and last week I forgot her name."
  Doctor: "Did you?"
  Patient: "Did I what?"
  Doctor: "Forget her name."
  Patient: "I'm not sure. I don't think so."
- Chronic substance abuse—In addition to using the popular street drugs, young people who cannot afford them will try sniffing gas, glue, or solvent from a plastic bag over their heads. They may die of asphyxiation if they lose consciousness before pulling the bag off. You may be asked to see one of these people after their first seizure. A short assessment of the patient's intellect will often reveal a wipeout of memory and thinking ability.
- Patients seen in a psychiatric ward or hospital or sent to you by a psychiatrist
- Patients who are said by a family member, themselves, or another physician to be depressed
- Patients with a major change in behavior, personality, dress, or **speech**

Irritability and frequent altercations with neighbors, coworkers, family, or the police over inconsequential issues, as well as faulty concentration, gross exaggeration in relating day-to-day activities, and a disinhibited attitude in a person with a previously rather careful approach to life may all signal the dementing process.

You will probably never see an unaccompanied patient who says, "Doctor, I'm losing my mind." It is almost axiomatic that as dementia advances, insight vanishes. The demented patient usually has no personal history and no physical signs.

Therefore, the history is dependent on the family member who spends the most time with the patient. The details needed include the patient's education level, occupation, hobbies, other illnesses, previous head injuries, seizures, and prescription and other drugs being taken.

Testing is done under the following headings: orientation, general information, memory, thinking (both abstract and logical), and calculation.

Orientation

Does the patient know the day, date, month, year, and time (within half an hour)? What is the name of the building he is now in, the city, province or state, and country? How did he get here—by car, bus, train, or trolley; from where and how long did it take? What is his full name, age, date of birth, and regimental number, if any? If he is an old soldier and the regimental number is forgotten, he is in serious trouble.

General Information

Every person carries a volume of information, some of which is a reflection of his own personal likes, hobbies, and habits. Ask the patient the name of the capital city of his country, how many provinces or states there are, who is the prime minister of Canada or the president of the United States, and the names of the past four prime ministers and the past four presidents— most Canadians seem to remember three Canadian prime ministers and five American presidents (it was ever thus). You can make up your own list of appropriate questions, having knowledge of the patient's premorbid occupation and interests as well as whatever is currently in the news.

Memory

There are three categories or stages of memory.

Immediate   Tell the patient you are about to give him

- A man's name
- The name of a flower
- A street address

Ask him to repeat them aloud as soon as he hears them. In about 3–5 min ask him to repeat the three items. Small degrees of dementia will interfere with this test.

Intermediate   Can the patient remember events that occurred yesterday or 1 week ago?

Remote   Does the patient know the names, ages, and dates of birth of his children; his own wedding date; his mother's maiden name; and such things as the dates of the beginning and end of World Wars I and II?

Thinking

Abstract   The interpretation of proverbs is a quick way to assess the ability of patients to think figuratively. Dementing patients think in literal, concrete ways. For example,

> Ask the patient the meaning of "A stitch in time saves nine."

The dementing person will talk about clothing, sewing, mending, and so on. The normal answer will be something about small amounts of early maintenance preventing major repairs at a later date.

Logical   Logical thinking can be tested with a variety of *short,* simple questions:

- What is similar between an orange and a lemon?
- What is similar between a pair of scissors and a knife?
- If you found a sealed, addressed, stamped envelope on the street, what would you do with it? *Correct:* Pick it up and drop it in the next mailbox. *Wrong:* Open it, find the name of the sender or the intended recipient, and try to contact one or the other, etc.

Calculation

Calculation is an inevitable part of all examinations of higher cerebral function. Difficulties with **numbers, words,** and **concentration** are among the most common presenting symptoms in dementia.

Number Recall

> Ask the patient to immediately repeat back to you a series of random, single-digit numbers.

Start with three numbers (eg, 7, 4, and 9), then four, and continue. Repetition by most people reveals recollection of seven digits forward and five backward. (This is a test more of concentration than of numerical skill, but it is a good way to start. Tests consisting of numbers seem to intimidate most people.)

100 Minus 7

> Ask the patient to subtract 7 from 100, to tell you the result, and then subtract 7 from 93, 7 from 86, and so on.

Most people can do this in about 90 s with no errors.

Miscellaneous Numerical and Concentration Tests

You can make your own tests. Generally, you are testing things learned by rote and the ability to manipulate information. Ask the patient,

- "How many 4¢ stamps can you get for a quarter [of a dollar]?"
- "What are 9 plus 3, 21 minus 8, 7 times 8, and 90 divided by 3?"
- "What is 7 times 2? Add 6 to the answer, divide that answer by 2, and subtract 3 from the answer. What number did you end with?"

A similar but less difficult test of concentration is to ask the patient to perform a multistep, consecutive act.

> Tell the patient "Stand up, pick up this piece of paper, face toward the window, and fold the paper."

The entire command is given before the patient starts.

Spatial and Constructional Ability

Defects in these functions may occur from disease in any part of the cerebrum on either side of the midline. However, parietal lobe lesions are most often the site, particularly if the rest of the cortical functions are more or less normal.

> Present the patient with consecutive drawings, one at a time, of two-dimensional or three-dimensional drawings and ask him to reproduce them.

If the patient has normal vision and a functioning dominant upper limb, he should be able to reproduce drawings like those in Figure 17–1, taking 1–1.5 min for each.

For more detailed methods of testing higher cerebral function, see *The Mental Status Examination in Neurology* (3rd ed., R.L. Strub and F.W. Black, editors. Davis, Philadelphia, 1993).

MOOD

Profound changes in mood are not a common part of organic neurological disease. There are exceptions. The dementing patient with insight will often

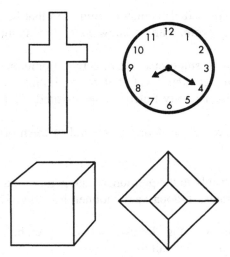

Figure 17–1. The patient with normal vision and function should be able to reproduce simple drawings like these in a relatively short period.

become depressed and thus compound his failing social and business abilities.

Endogenous depression with normal intellectual ability may mimic dementia. Euphoria and emotional lability may be part of intrinsic brain stem disease as well as a drug response.

Early morning wakening, loss of interest, chronic fatigue, diminished appetite, irritability, impotence, and frigidity are all common manifestations of depression. Some patients eat to excess when depressed. Do not hesitate to ask patients whether they are depressed, do they cry, do they feel like crying, or does music or a sentimental story bring them to the verge of tears?

The cyclothymic, manic-depressive patient with organic disease presents a challenge. In the down phase of his cycle he is negative about everything, his answers are rather limited, and little is volunteered. In the manic phase he is an unstoppable talker with difficulty staying on the subject.

DISEASES OF INTELLECT AND MEMORY

Delirium

Delirium is a state of confusion and amnesia of recent onset. One must assume that it is diagnosable and treatable and should act accordingly.

The patient is confused. This may be minor, in that he does not know the date or the time, or severe, with no knowledge of his name, the place, or any other identifying facts.

He may be drowsy, stuporous or overactive, tremulous, and agitated. He may be hallucinating at either level of alertness. Eating, rest and sleep, washing, and the details of bodily functions are ignored. Epileptic seizures may occur.

There are many causes of delirium; several of them originate outside the central nervous system.

- *Infections:* Commonly in the pulmonary and genitourinary tracts
- *Drugs:* Barbiturates, L-dopa, anticholinergics, steroids, and anesthetic agents
- *Hypoxia:* Obstructive lung disease, pulmonary embolus, myocardial infarct, and congestive heart failure
- *Metabolic:* Lung, liver, or kidney failure; hyponatremia; hyperglycemia; alcohol withdrawal; and postoperative electrolyte imbalance
- *Central nervous system diseases:* Postictal state, subarachnoid hemorrhage, head injury, cerebral thromboses, encephalitis, meningitis, and brain abscess

The diagnosis and management of acute delirium call for energetic and wide-ranging thinking by the attending doctor.

Meningitis does not always cause a stiff neck in the elderly; pneumonia may not raise body temperature or change the white blood cell count.

The mildly demented elderly man may have quite a passable existence at home with familiar surroundings, pets, and family. One night in the hospital for a single cataract operation under local anesthetic may change him into a frightened, hallucinating, overactive, delirious person. When he returns to his preadmission state within 1 day of being home but was amnesic for all of his hospital stay, we realize how fragile is the stability of the central nervous system.

Dementia

Dementia is failure of the intellect, which often starts as a subtle decay in social graces and business abilities. The conduct and behavior changes may combine or alternate with impulsiveness or apathy. Judgment, initiative, and decision making become blunted. Memory deficits eventually become the dominant problem. These deficits are initially for new information and recent memory, but the amnesic process extends backward into the earlier parts of the patient's life. Confabulatory stories often fill the patient's conversation. A stranger can be completely taken in with the glib and resourceful verbal inventions of the demented.

Speech disturbances, word-finding difficulties, anomia, and other dysphasic signs are common. Depression and agitation are equally common. The demented person may forget or refuse to eat, spend the night pacing the floor, and ignore personal hygiene.

The process can begin at age 40. Inability to remember the names of friends is so common at age 40–50 that it is normal. The rate of progression is variable although difficult to assess accurately because the onset is subtle and not clearly identified. Most demented patients incapable of caring for themselves are in their sixth or seventh decade. Relatives usually say that the patient's memory and intellect have been slipping for the previous 4–5 years, but it has been much more obvious in the immediate 6 months. The disease does not accelerate, but when basic skills needed for dressing, washing, eating, and other activities of daily living have vanished, the process appears to be more acute.

Dementia is always organic, is almost always progressive, and is rarely treatable. The common causes are

- Alzheimer's disease—Diagnosed by exclusion of other diseases; can be proven only histologically
- Normal-pressure hydrocephalus—See Chapter 12.
- Huntington's chorea, supranuclear palsy, parkinsonism, spinocerebellar degeneration, and Jakob-Creutzfeld disease
- Meningioma, glioma, abscess, subdural hematoma, postmeningitis or encephalitis, and general paresis
- Hypoxia, hypoglycemia, head injury, and multiple cerebral infarctions
- Pernicious anemia, hypothyroidism, chronic renal failure, chronic dialysis, Wilson's disease, pellagra, and Wernicke-Korsakoff syndrome

As in the management of a patient with acute delirium, the physician must be thorough and thoughtful in the investigation of the demented patient. The family needs help and support, and the patient needs protection. If a treatable lesion cannot be found, this must be faced and the inevitability of the disease process must be explained. If the patient can be cared for at home without exhausting the spouse, this is probably the best arrangement. Eventually, institutional care will be necessary.

Disorders of Speech 18

Aphasia is a loss or impairment of language caused by disease of the cerebrum. In this sense, *language* means "speaking, writing, reading, and listening." The words *aphasia* and *dysphasia* are used interchangeably.

The parkinsonian patient with low-amplitude, monotone, arrhythmic speech or the patient with cerebellar disease and staccato speech are not aphasic; they are **dysarthric**. The patient with bilateral vocal cord paresis is **aphonic**. Stammering or stuttering is not aphasia. Some psychotic or demented patients repeat whatever is said to them. This is **echolalia**, and in these patients it is not part of aphasia.

The acute schizophrenic may have a fluent, unintelligible jumble of words and neologisms. This is part of his **thought disorder**, not aphasia.

Finally, the patient who is **mute** because of psychosis or other reasons cannot be said to be aphasic. He may be, but you cannot say so.

Anatomy
Language is a function of the *dominant* cerebral hemisphere. Most people are right-handed, and their left hemisphere is dominant. Of the 5–10% who are left-handed, the majority also have a dominant left hemisphere.

- *Broca's area:* This is Brodmann's area 44 at the posterior end of the third frontal convolution and is concerned with the **motor** aspects of language.
- *Wernicke's area:* This is Brodmann's areas 41 and 42 at the posterior end of the superior temporal gyrus. Deep to Wernicke's area in the insula are the transverse gyri of Heschl. These are the **primary** auditory cortices. These areas are concerned with understanding **spoken** language.
- *Angular gyrus:* This is Brodmann's area 39 and surrounds the terminal vertical part of the superior temporal sulcus. It is part of the important inferior parietal lobule. It is concerned with the understanding of **written** language.
- *Supramarginal gyrus:* Brodmann's area 40 surrounds the terminal vertical end of the lateral sulcus and is the other part of the inferior parietal lobule. It is also concerned with the comprehension of language.

These cortical areas are connected to each other and to other cortical areas by the **arcuate fasciculus**. They also have connections to the thalamus and the nondominant cerebral hemisphere. These anatomical areas concerned with language each have an associated type of speech disorder, for example, Broca's area and an expressive aphasia, or Wernicke's area and a receptive aphasia. This is simplistic. Clinically, patients do not display sharply defined and distinctive dysphasias that are exclusively defects of expression or defects of reception. A Broca's aphasia, for example, if the result of a small superficial lesion, can present with defects of spoken and written speech only. A lesion in the same cortical area, but deeper, will produce the same defects plus defects of comprehension.

All areas of the brain concerned with language are supplied by the middle cerebral artery. There are many reports of normal language with disease in these areas, although the reverse is not true. The areas are not cytologically distinctive, and electrical stimulation of them in the awake patient has not revealed great information.

Language should be thought of as a combined function of some primary sensory or motor areas in concert with their appropriate association areas plus the white matter fasciculi connecting them.

EXAMINATION OF THE APHASIC PATIENT

Spontaneous Speech
Fluency is the most important thing to note about the patient's spontaneous speech.

Fluent Speech
In fluent speech the words pour forth, paraphasia, neologisms, and errors included. *Nonfluent* means that the patient has few words; he labors with pursed lips and much frustration, then brings out three words after 10 s of trying. Also note the content, comprehensiveness, and errors.

Repetition
Ask the patient to repeat words, numbers, and sentences. Keep your speech slow, regular, and loud. The two most helpful tests in assessing an aphasic patient are **fluency** and **ability to repeat**.

Comprehension
Ask the patient to perform some act that verifies his understanding of spoken speech, for example, "Point to the door," "Touch your ear," "Stand up," "Sit down," or "Is today Wednesday?" (the patient's head nod or shake being used as a "yes" or "no" response).

Some conflicts may occur here—a defect of body image or an apraxia may prevent the patient from pointing to his ear or another part of his body, confusion may cause the wrong answer to the day-of-the-week question, and a disorder of language is not the cause of their error. Also, if your questions are too close together, the answer to the last question may be used for the next question. This is **perseveration** and is not diagnostic, being present to a greater or lesser extent in almost all types of aphasias.

Naming

Ask the patient to name familiar, everyday objects. Go slowly and start with big, whole objects and then the smaller parts of objects. A patient may have normal naming ability for "watch," "strap," and "buckle," but when you point to the stem, hands, or numerals of the watch, he is lost and tries to describe these smaller parts by their function, for example, "the thing you wind it with."

Reading

Give the patient some simple thing to read aloud. Write short, one-step commands that you wish him to read and obey in order to test his comprehension for written language. Some types of aphasia show excellent comprehension of written material but a major defect in reading aloud.

Writing

Ask the patient to write a spontaneous sentence or dictate a sentence for her. Her signature is not suitable.

TYPES OF APHASIA

Broca's Aphasia

This lesion is in Broca's area and its deep white matter connections. This is a disorder of language **output**.

The patient is **nonfluent** and cannot repeat, name, read aloud, or write. He usually can understand written and spoken language, although, if stressed by repeated commands given quickly, defects can be shown here also. The patient may have only two or three words that are used over and over or he may burst out with profanities while attempting to speak. He looks and acts frustrated by his illness. Weakness and sensory loss of the right lower face, arm, and leg are frequent accompaniments. In recovery, the speech remains slow and agonizing, lacks rhythm and finesse, and is made up mostly of nouns or isolated verbs.

Wernicke's Aphasia

This lesion is in Wernicke's area, and this is a sensory or receptive disorder.

The patient is fluent and cannot repeat, name, read aloud, comprehend writing, or write. Unlike those with Broca's dysphasia, the patient with the posterior lesion is a relaxed, comfortable, voluble talker. The sentences are devoid of meaning. They are filled with neologisms and paraphasias. The rhythm is more or less normal, and the length of phrases and sentences often seems normal. There is some hesitation and searching for words, but nothing like the lockjawed consternation of the patient with Broca's lesion.

The patient cannot hear himself and usually shows no concern over his jargon of scrambled words and near-words. Some patients have a greater defect in understanding spoken speech as opposed to written speech, while the reverse may be present in others.

A hemiparesis is an *uncommon* accompaniment of this type of aphasia, as is a cerebral sensory defect. Quadrantanopic field defects are more likely to be found.

Conduction Aphasia

This lesion is in the arcuate fasciculus that connects Broca's and Wernicke's areas.

The patient is **fluent** and can comprehend what he reads and hears, but cannot repeat, name, read aloud, or write. There are many pauses and word searches, and the fluency is less than in Wernicke's dysphasia. The patient can hear his errors and paraphasias and often has better performance once he has started or is into a sequence of words (eg, counting). The patient understands what he hears and reads but can repeat neither.

Anomic Aphasia

This is also known as amnesic and nominal aphasia. It is not related to a single local lesion.

The patient is fluent, but has trouble finding words. She has pauses, substitutions, and much circuitous, meaningless speech. This is evident in spontaneous speech and in naming. All other aspects of language except writing may be normal.

Anomic aphasia is present, to a greater or lesser degree, in all aphasias. It is the most common residual defect after any aphasia.

Global Aphasia

This lesion is large, involving both Broca's and Wernicke's areas. All aspects of language function are abnormal. The patients are nonfluent, and all tests of language are abnormal. Global aphasia is commonly accompanied by hemiparesis, hemisensory loss, and a hemianopia.

OTHER LANGUAGE DISORDERS

Sensory and motor transcortical aphasias, pure word deafness, pure word blindness (alexia) with and without agraphia, pure word muteness (aphemia), and thalamic and striatal aphasia are outside the scope of this work.

Suggested Additional Reading

Rose, F. Clifford and Whurr, Renata: *Aphasia*. Whurr Publishers Ltd, United Kingdom, 2000.

Basso, Anna: *Aphasia and Its Therapy*. Oxford University Press, Oxford, New York, 2003.

Zaidel, Eran and Iacoboni, Marco: *The Parallel Brain*. MIT Press, Cambridge, MA, 2003.

Appendix: *Neurological Examination Instruments*

All kinds of instruments are available. They vary in price, and some are associated with the great ancient heroes of European and British neurology.

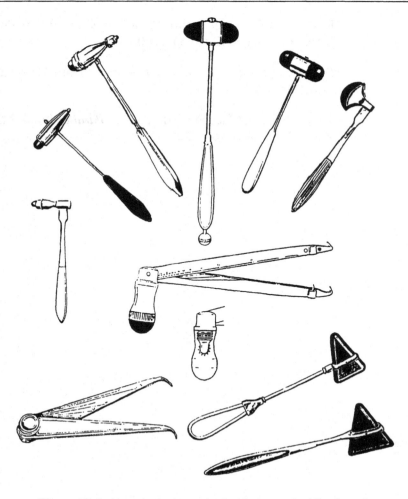

Figure 18–1. Neurological examination instruments. (*Continued*)

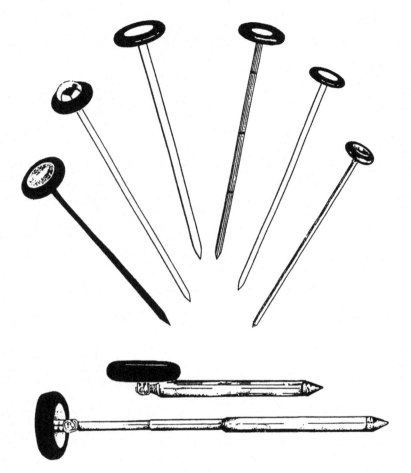

Figure 18–1 (continued). Neurological examination instruments.

The cheapest reflex hammer works exactly the same as the most expensive; the cheapest 128 tuning fork is all you need for examining one aspect of posterior column function. Do not buy an instrument for testing pain sensation. A package of sterile pins is all you need. Each patient is examined with his own pin that is then discarded. The instruments in Figure 18–1 can be bought from Kennex Medical Inc., PO Box 870009, Stone Mountain, GA 30087.

Index

NOTE: Page numbers in bold face type indicate a major discussion. A *t* following a page number indicates tabular material and an *f* following a page number indicates a figure.